A-Z Notes in Radiological Practice and Reporting

W0228170

Series Editors

Carlo N. De Cecco
Department of Radiology and Radiological Sciences,
Medical University of South Carolina,
Charleston, SC, USA

Andrea Laghi
Department of Radiological Sciences, Oncology
and Pathology, Sapienza - University of Rome,
Rome, Italy

The new series A-Z notes in Radiological Practice and Reporting provides practical guides for residents and general radiologists, organized alphabetically, primarily according to disease or condition. All booklets are designed so as to comprise only a small number of illustrations and to cover a large spectrum of topics referring to different anatomical regions of interest. Entries typically include a short description of pathological and clinical characteristics, guidance on selection of the most appropriate imaging technique, a schematic review of potential diagnostic clues, and useful tips and tricks.

- Useful in daily practice for planning exams and radiologic reporting
- Quick answer to frequent questions occurring during daily radiological practice
- Practical and brief notes organized in the form of an A-Z glossary
- Easy and fast consultation

More information about this series at
http://www.springer.com/series/11569

Marcello Osimani • Claudio Chillemi

Knee Imaging

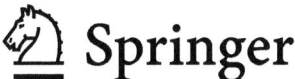 Springer

Marcello Osimani
Department of Radiological
Sciences, Oncology
and Pathology
Sapienza University of Rome
Latina
Italy

Claudio Chillemi
Department of Orthopaedics
and Traumatology
Istituto Chirurgico Ortopedico
Traumatologico (ICOT)
Latina
Italy

ISSN 2284-2616   ISSN 2284-3884   (electronic)
A-Z Notes in Radiological Practice and Reporting
ISBN 978-88-470-3949-0   ISBN 978-88-470-3950-6   (eBook)
DOI 10.1007/978-88-470-3950-6

Library of Congress Control Number: 2016954023

This Springer imprint is published by Springer Nature
The registered company is Springer-Verlag Italia Srl.

Foreword

The volume "Knee Imaging" was drawn up by Dr. Marcello Osimani, an expert musculoskeletal Radiologist. Across a simple lecture, the reader is able to deepen, in a complete way, some imaging signs that are critical for the correct identification and comprehension of various knee joint pathologies. In this manner, not only the correct imaging technique and interpretation for an accurate reporting of articular lesions were taken into account, but the differential diagnosis and some specific aspects that may create difficulties are especially well represented. Specific attention was paid to all those conditions that can mimic different diseases in order to avoid under- or over-estimation of the actual articular pathology. A complete and high-quality iconography was inserted and deeply analyzed. The assessment of minimal lesions and the coupling between the iconographic aspects and correct diagnostic interpretation were also highlighted using the different radiological signs.

This book is easy to understand and best suited for a daily practical use or quick reference.

Carlo Masciocchi

Foreword to This Series

A-Z Notes in Radiological Practice and Reporting is a new series of practical guides dedicated to residents and general radiologists. The series was born thanks to the original idea to bring to the public attention a series of notes collected by doctors and fellows during their clinical activity and attendance at international academic institutions. Those brief notes were critically reviewed, sometimes integrated, cleaned up, and organized in the form of an A-Z glossary to be usable by a third reader

The ease and speed of consultation and the agility in reading were behind the construction of this series and were the reasons why the booklets are organized alphabetically, primarily according to disease or condition. The number of illustrations has been deliberately reduced and focused only on those ones relevant to the specific entry. Residents and general radiologists will find in these booklets numerous quick answers to frequent questions occurring during radiological practice, which will be useful in daily activity for planning exams and radiological reporting.

Each single entry typically includes a short description of pathological and clinical characteristics, guidance on selection of the most appropriate imaging technique, a schematic review of potential diagnostic clues, and useful tips and tricks.

This series will include the most relevant topics in radiology, starting with cardiac imaging and continuing with the gastrointestinal tract, liver, pancreas and bile ducts, and genitourinary apparatus during the first 2 years. More arguments will be covered in the next issues.

The editors put a lot of their efforts in selecting the most appropriate colleagues willing to exchange with readers their own experiences in their respective fields. The result is a combination of experienced professors, enthusiastic researchers, and young talented radiologists working together within a single framework project with the primary aim of making their knowledge available for residents and general practitioners.

We really do hope that this series can meet the satisfaction of the readers and can help them in their daily radiological practice.

Charleston, USA   Carlo N. De Cecco
Rome, Italy   Andrea Laghi

Acknowledgment

Special Thanks for editing to:

Marta Zerunian, MD

Department of Radiological Sciences, Oncology and Pathology

University of Rome "Sapienza" – Polo Pontino, Latina, Italy

Luca Bertana, MD

Department of Radiological Sciences, Oncology and Pathology

University of Rome "Sapienza" – Polo Pontino, Latina, Italy

Abbreviations

ACL	Anterior cruciate ligament
AP	Anterior-posterior
BLOKS	Boston-Leeds Osteoarthritis Knee Score
BMLs	Subchondral bone marrow lesions
CT	Computed tomography
CUBE	Is not an acronym. This is the corresponding GE vendor acronym for Siemens SPACE sequence
DESS	Dual echo steady state
dGEMRIC	Delayed gadolinium-enhanced MRI of cartilage
FOV	Field of view
FS	Fat saturation
FSE	Fast spin echo
GAGs	Glucosaminoglycans
Gd	Gadolinium
GRE	Gradient-recalled echo
ITB	Iliotibial band
LL	Latero-lateral
LM	Lateral meniscus
MCL	Medial collateral ligament
MCS	Meniscocapsular separation
MFLs	Meniscofemoral ligaments
MFPL	Medial femoral-patellar ligaments
MM	Medial meniscus

MOAKS	Magnetic Resonance Osteoarthritis Knee Score
MOCART	Magnetic resonance observations of cartilage repair tissue
MPR	Multiplanar reconstruction
OA	Osteoarthritis
OCD	Osteochondritis dissecans
OSs	Osgood-Schlatter syndrome
PCL	Posterior cruciate ligament
PD	Proton density
PLC	Posterolateral corner of the knee
PMC	Posteromedial corner of the knee
PPV	Positive predictive value
ROI	Region of interest
SALTR	Acronym for slipped, above, lower, through/transverse/together, ruined/rammed in Salter-Harris fractures
SH	Salter-Harris
SNR	Signal-to-noise ratio
SPACE	Sampling perfection with application-optimized contrasts using different flip angle evolution
SPGR	Spoiled gradient recalled acquisition in the steady state
SSFP	Steady-state free precession
TE	Echo time
TR	Repetition time
TSE	Turbo spin echo
TT-TG	Tibial tubercle to trochlear groove
VIPR	Vastly interpolated projection reconstruction
VISTA	Volumetric isotropic T2w acquisition
VR	Volume rendering
WORMS	Whole-Organ MR Imaging Score

Contents

A

Ahlbäck Classification System

Classification for grading knee osteoarthritis. It must be performed on plain weight-bearing AP radiographs.

It is possible to divide the alterations in five grades according to severity: (1) joint rim space <3 mm, (2) rim disappearance, (3) subchondral sclerosis and remodeling (0–5 mm), (4) subchondral sclerosis and remodeling (5–10 mm), and (5) severe subchondral sclerosis and remodeling (>10 mm) with joint axis alterations.

AIIS Avulsion Injury

The AIIS represents the proximal attachment of the extensor mechanism. It is important to know that the rectus femoris tendon is the most involved tendon on quadriceps injuries, both by flexion of the hip and extension of the knee, and has two branches of insertion, first on AIIS and a second on the hip capsule called indirect or reflected tendon. On MR images, attention must be reserved also on the hip when AIIS and rectus femoris edema is seen.

M. Osimani, C. Chillemi, *Knee Imaging*, A-Z Notes in Radiological Practice and Reporting, DOI 10.1007/978-88-470-3950-6_1, © Springer-Verlag Italia 2017

Anterior Cruciate Ligament, Anatomy

The anterior cruciate ligament (ACL) is an oblique extra-synovial ligament that courses in the intercondylar groove, from the anterior area of the proximal tibial plate to the medial facet of the lateral femoral condyle. It has two fiber bundles, the anteromedial and the posteromedial, and, occasionally, a third bundle between these two bundles.

The ACL measures more or less 40 mm in length and 13 mm in width.

Anterior Cruciate Ligament, Acute Tear MR Imaging

MRI

ACL tear must be evaluated both with primary signs and secondary or associated signs on MR images.

- *Primary signs*: ligament rupture involves a change of the signal intensity of the fibers and their morphological and anatomical course.

- Although the oblique sagittal plane is considered as the most helpful in diagnosis, we prefer to use the axial plane as the main plane, avoiding magic angle artifact, with the support of coronal and sagittal imaging. In the acute phase, the ligament appears thickened and fibers show high signal intensity in T2- or intermediate-weighted sequences. As the blood vessels of ACL are located between longitudinal fiber bundles, high signal on T1-weighted images has to be interpreted as a tear of almost one-half of the ligament, resulting in blood infarction (ill-defined area of focal edema and hemorrhage) (Fig. 1). The aspects must be distinguished from

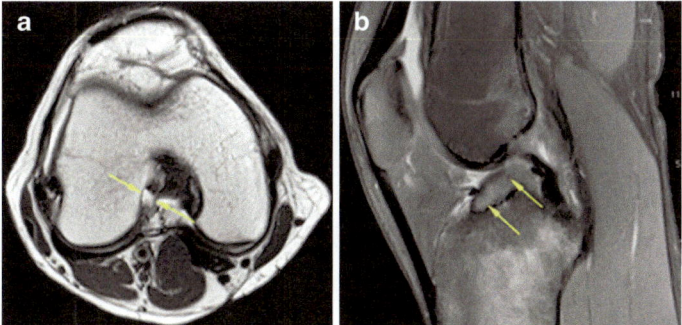

Figure 1 ACL complete disruption: axial T2-weighted image (**a**) shows fibers interruption with fluid on the ligament (*arrows* in **a**); on (**b**) sagittal PD FS image, the ligament appears deflected with enlarged shape (*arrows* in **b**)

mucoid degeneration of the intact ACL (see relative lemma). The ACL ligament should be considered disrupted when its course has the long axis more horizontal than Blumensaat line: a line projected along the intercondylar roof (see lemma) on sagittal images.

- *Secondary signs*: several signs associated with articular lesions probably correlated with the injure mechanism. These have low sensitivity, but the presence of secondary signs should lead us to seek ACL abnormalities or associated crucial meniscal or capsular lesions. The main classified signs are (see lemmas) (1) bone bruise, pivot shift, (2) femorotibial translation, (3) Segond fracture, (4) arched-appearing PCL, and (5) deep lateral femoral notch sign.

Anterior Cruciate Ligament, Ganglion

Anterior cruciate ligament cysts may be differentiated in intra-ligamentous and extraligamentous ganglions.

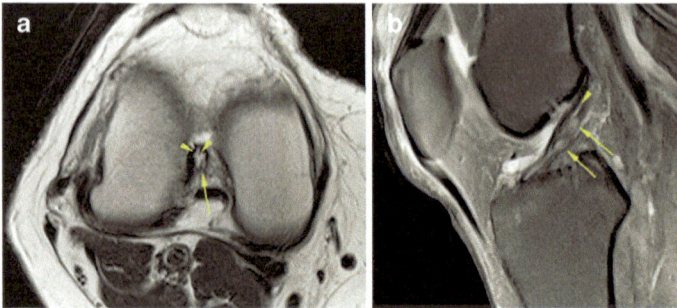

Figure 2 ACL ganglia: axial T2-weighted image (**a**) shows peripheral fibers interruption (*arrows*) with fluid on the ligament (*arrowhead*); on (**b**) sagittal PD FS, cystic fluid collection with intermediate signal may be seen on the ligament (*arrows*)

The most common is the extraligamentous location and appears like a synovial recess but well defined, often septated near the ACL. Fibers or intrasubstance ganglions of ACL are less common; their identification becomes crucial as ACL ganglions can be difficult to appreciate on standard arthroscopy; therefore, on the basis of MRI diagnosis, the arthroscopist may decide to probe the ACL or add a posterior portal. On MRI, cyst appears similar to a partial tear, but unlike the latter, it is oriented parallel to the long axis of the ligament with a concomitant normal-appearing ACL (Figs. 2 and 3).

Anterior Cruciate Ligament, Imaging Technical Features

• *Radiography*: Radiographs have a limited significance in the evaluation of bone indirect signs of ACL injury. On radiographs or on computed tomography (CT), avulsion bone fractures at the tibial or femoral insertion have to be reported. Segond fracture is a type of avulsion fracture of the iliotibial

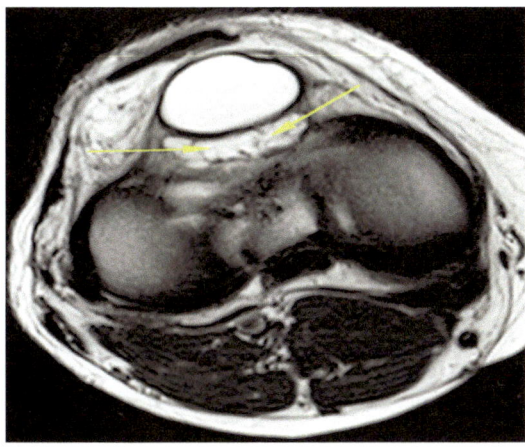

Figure 3 Intra-articular ganglion cysts: axial T2-weighted image shows capsulated cystic lesion within the infrapatellar Hoffa's fat pad. Note the displacement of the anterior intermeniscal ligament (lateral aspect of the cyst) and the absent communication with ACL or menisci (*arrows*)

band on the lateral tibial plate (see lemma Segond fracture) and is commonly related with an ACL tear. As result of osteochondral impaction, a fracture may be appreciated on the lateral femoral condyle (lateral femoral notch sign) as sulcus deeper than 1.5 mm. Opacity on suprapatellar recess may be a sign of hemarthrosis that is very common in ACL injuries.

- *Computed tomography*: Computed tomography (CT) may be helpful in the better depiction of avulsion fracture, above all with three-dimensional reconstruction I in the presurgical phase.
- *Magnetic resonance*: MRI has the most important role in the detection of ACL injury because of high accuracy in excluding a tear. Protocol has to be performed above all for optimal demonstration of associated meniscus and cartilage disruptions as a protocol that images the menisci and cartilage optimally also show ACL injures. Although ACL is optimally

assessed with the knee in about 30–40° of flexion, flexion makes arduous the correct evaluation of the menisci and other knee ligaments. The normal anterior cruciate fibers appear as low to intermediate signal intensity parallel to the intercondylar line. The ligament has to be taut in all planes (both axial) and sequences. The low signal is related to a decreased proton mobility in the fibers and dephasing of hydrogen nuclei that results in T2 shortening. The minimal protocol requirements of ACL imaging include 2D fast spin echo T2-weighted sequences (or proton-weighted fat suppressed) in 2–3 orthogonal planes. Different planes (e.g., axial plane) may be used for anatomical correlation, above all when increased signal intensity seen in ligaments and tendons is related to internal degeneration, or probably magic-angle artifact and patients malpositioning. In our center, the standard knee protocol includes a coronal T2-weighted or PD fat-suppressed sequence, TSE sagittal T1-weighted sequence, and TSE axial intermediate-weighted or PD with fat-suppression sequence. T1-weighted sequences are helpful for evaluation of menisci, suspected fracture, or loose bodies. Some centers perform oblique parasagittal views, slightly oblique no more than 10° off perpendicular, along the ACL; we do not perform this additional sequence because we prefer to follow the ligament in a different plane. In some difficult or uncertain case (internal disruption or ganglion), we perform a 3D FSE imaging with or without FS, because the thinner slice thickness permits to show fluid relation with the ligament.

Anterior Cruciate Ligament, Chronic Tear Imaging

In chronic phase of an ACL tear, as the fibrous involution become prominent on the edema, it is possible to notice a thin low-signal intensity on periligamentous synovial course or a "serpiginous" ligament or even an empty notch sign on coronal imaging. This aspect may produce a low-signal nodule similar to cyclops lesion in the postoperative ACL ("pseudo-cyclops" appearance).

Bone bruise is less evident than in the acute phase, but osteochondral lesions may be excluded (see chondral imaging).

Anterior Cruciate Ligament, Mucoid Degeneration

This represents a process of senescent degeneration of the ligament, and MRI appearances may mimic a partial ACL tear. The ACL is enlarged with proximal areas with increased signal without fluid-like appearance, and the ligament on sagittal planes is similar to a "celery stalk." Higher signal intensity in T1- and T2-weighted images is due to mucoid matrix in the ACL; this condition may be differentiated from a partial tear on the basis of non-traumatic history, a negative Lachman test, and the absence of secondary signs of an ACL tear. Clinical symptoms may include pain, swelling symptoms, and mechanical locking.

Anterior Cruciate Ligament, Partial Tear

Partial tears are more difficult to assess in MRI because changes in signal and morphology are less evident. A partial tear may be suspected when linear hyperintensity through the fibers is associated with quite deflection of the ligament (like a hammock). These signs have a sensitivity (40–75 %) and specificity (51–89 %), depending on MRI field (better on 3 Tesla scanners) (Fig. 4).

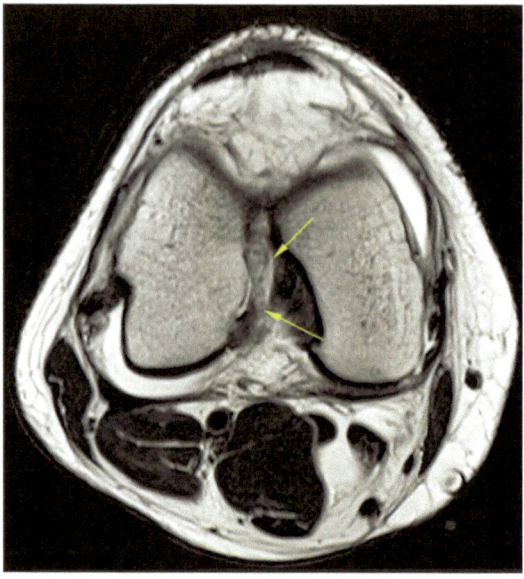

Figure 4 ACL partial lesion: T2-weighted TSE image shows a hyperintense ACL with elongated morphology of residual fibers (*arrows*)

Anterior Cruciate Ligament, Post-surgery Imaging

Femoral and tibial tunnel correct positioning: a correct femoral tunnel is the main aspect in maintaining graft isometry, while a correct tibial tunnel is the primary factor in preventing impingement of the graft against the roof of the intercondylar notch.

- *Radiographs or coronal and sagittal MRI* must be evaluated for assessment of correct positioning of the tunnels. The femoral tunnel should be located at the intersection of a line on the posterior cortex of the femur and another line along the roof of the intercondylar notch (lateral radiograph or sagittal

MR images) and should open at the superolateral posterior margin of the intercondylar notch (anteroposterior radiograph or coronal MR images). The tibial tunnel should be oriented parallel to the Blumensaat line (see lemma), and it should be possible to follow the intra-articular opening of the tunnel until the Blumensaat line meets the tibial tuberosity.

- *Graft MRI characteristics*: MRI evaluation of ACL graft should be performed after 4–8 months from the surgery, because of the signal becoming normally low on short-TE sequences and usually completely resolving by 12 months. The increased signal must be evaluated and should be due to abnormal graft revascularization and synovialization. When semitendinosus and gracilis tendon are used as graft, a fluid signal on T2-weighted images should be normal as the graft is composed by four strands. A tear of the graft is perpendicular on the long axis of the graft, while normal fluid between the fibers is parallel.
- *Graft tear*: graft tear is more frequent in the remodeling phase from 4 to 12 months after surgery. Graft tear must be suspected especially on axial T2 images, when an increased persistent signal, thickness, or fiber discontinuity is seen. Anterior tibial translation and an exposed posterior horn of the lateral meniscus are secondary signs helpful for distinguishing the graft hyperintensity for revascularization process from a tear. Fiber discontinuity must be evaluated also in sagittal or coronal planes. When a posterior bowing of the graft is seen, a "graft stretching" in the clinical setting of increased laxity must be suspected.
- *Graft impingement*: a tibial tunnel malpositioned too anterior on radiography, CT, and MRI is the first aspect affecting a graft impingement on the roof of the intercondylar notch. Signal changes of the graft on MRI are more focal unlike the revascularization and persist beyond a year. As the impingement may lead to graft rupture, contacts with the bone must be evaluated for arthroscopic notchplasty.

- *Arthrofibrosis*: the nodular form appears as low-signal "cyclops lesion" on the distal end of the graft, between the femur and tibia. The fibrosis may also spread and involve the Hoffa's fat pad and may expand to synovial layers with capsule thickening.

• *Intra-articular bodies*: when there is suspicion of a cartilage or a cortical bone fragment mostly in the intercondylar notch, gradient-echo sequences must be performed in order to assess the cortical as low-signal intensity. Patellar synovial recess must be also evaluated for bone or chondral fragment, overlooked during the procedure or primary misdiagnosed.

• *Cystic degeneration*: it is similar to the ganglion of the native ACL, but the fluid collection may spread along the tunnel portion of the graft or distally into the soft tissues anterior to the tibial tubercle. The signal of the tunnels must be carefully evaluated, because a pressure rise due to the fluid in the graft may cause an enlargement of the tunnel for bone remodeling with fixation failure or mobilization. While a linear fluid collection may be normal with doubled gracilis semitendinosus graft, it is abnormal with patellar tendon. A graft tear appears more focal without inner intact fiber in the fluid (Fig. 5).

Arcuate Ligament Complex

This complex includes the lateral collateral ligament; the biceps femoris tendon; the popliteus tendon; the popliteomeniscal and popliteofibular ligaments; oblique popliteal, fabellofibular ligaments; and lateral gastrocnemius muscle. These structures are difficult to assess on a standard plane for a MRI knee protocol. When an ACL disruption is seen, an oblique coronal plane parallel to the popliteus tendon may be helpful to exclude a concomitant posterior-lateral damage (Fig. 6).

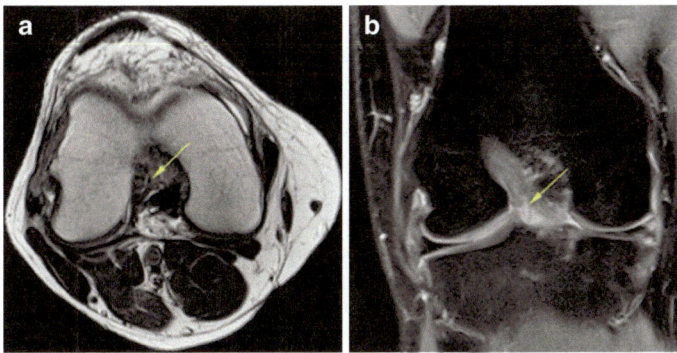

Figure 5 Failed ACL graft: images of axial T2-weighted (**a**) and coronal PD FS (**b**) show graft enlargement, signal dishomogeneity, and absent fibers (*arrow* in **a** and **b**)

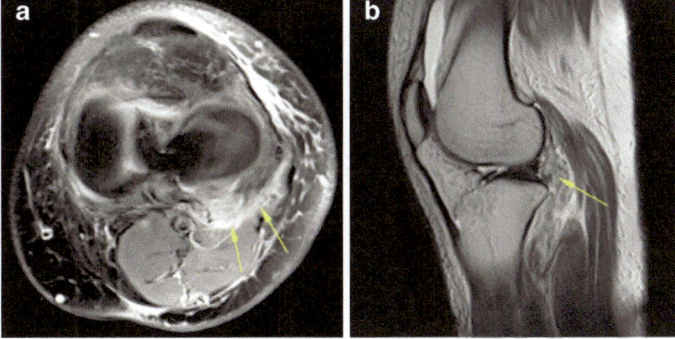

Figure 6 Arcuate ligament complex tear: images (**a** and **b**) show abnormal signal and morphology of popliteus muscle (*arrows* in **a** and **b**) with large tear of the posterolateral capsule (note that popliteus tendon and popliteomeniscal ligament in b are not visible)

Arcuate Complex Avulsion Fracture

The arcuate ligament complex is one of the stabilizers of the knee and is composed by several structures including arcuate, fabellofibular, and popliteofibular ligaments. The identification of these injuries is crucial in terms of knee stability considering it's correlated with other stabilizers injuries as well as ACL and can influence the outcome of ACL reconstruction.

- *Radiography*: the image of the avulsed fracture, including shape and size, varies according to which ligaments are involved. The avulsed bone fragment is simply identified by AP oblique view with internal rotation as an elliptic piece of bone arising from the fibular styloid process with long axis oriented horizontally "arcuate sign." Visualization on the lateral view may be limited by its superimposition over the posterior tibia.
- *MRI*: MR imaging may clarify soft tissue component of the injury, confirming the exact origin of the fracture fragments, either by identification of marrow edema in the head of the fibula and any soft-tissue swelling next to the injury. An MRI may help to evaluate commonly associated injuries such as cruciate ligament injuries, lateral capsular ligament, collateral ligaments, popliteus muscle, and meniscal tears.

Suggested Reading

Hernández-Vaquero D et al (2012) Relationship between radiological grading and clinical status in knee osteoarthritis. A multicentric study. BMC Musculoskelet Disord 13:194

Papalia R, Torre G, Vasta S et al (2015) Bone bruises in anterior cruciate ligament injured knee and long-term outcomes. A review of the evidence. Open Access J Sports Med 6:37–48

Wright RW (2014) Osteoarthritis classification scales: interobserver reliability and arthroscopic correlation. J Bone Joint Surg Am 96(14):1145–1151

B

Blumensaat Line

Line projected along the intercondylar roof on sagittal knee images. It may be used for the evaluation of correct alignment of tibial tunnel after ACL reconstruction or in the assessment of deflected ligament after ACL injuries.

Bone Bruise, Pivot Shift

A bone bruise related to ACL injury is commonly caused by osseous impact during pivot-shift rotatory mechanisms in which there is external rotation of the lateral condyle relative to the fixed tibia. Medullary signal becomes high on T2-weighted images due to osseous edema, subcortical microfracture, or hemorrhage (Fig. 1). When anteromedial mechanism is prevalent, the bone bruise is located more frequently in the posteromedial tibial plateau, near the semimembranosus tendon insertion. According to our experience, bone bruising is considered a sign of ACL tear (highly likely near 90%), except in pediatric or adolescent patients with more elastic ligament.

M. Osimani, C. Chillemi, *Knee Imaging*, A-Z Notes in Radiological Practice and Reporting, DOI 10.1007/978-88-470-3950-6_2, © Springer-Verlag Italia 2017

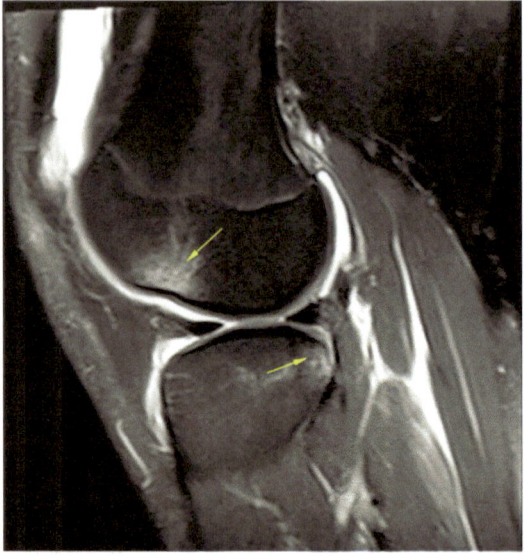

Figure 1 Bone bruise: sagittal PD FS image shows hyperintense areas on the anterior aspect of the femur and on the posterior aspect of the tibia (*arrows*), suggesting a bone impact during pivot shift

Bosch-Bock Bump

It is a protruding osseous excrescence located 2–5 mm below the lateral articular margin of the tibia. This should be a sign of a chronic tear of the ACL.

Bucket-Handle Tear

A bucket-handle tear is defined as a longitudinal tear with displacement of the "handle" fragment (Fig. 2) more frequent in MM. Various MR signs were proposed (sensitive but not spe-

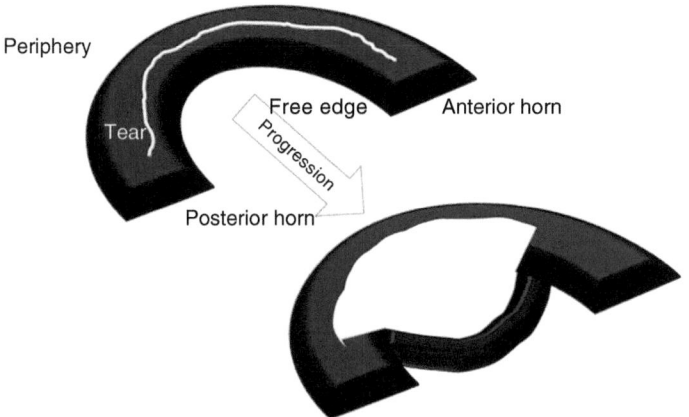

Figure 2 The scheme represents a bucket-handle tear. This is the evolution of a large longitudinal tear with displacement of the "handle" fragment

cific): the absence of bow tie (longitudinal tear breach), a fragment within the intercondylar notch, a double PCL (fragment displaced under the PCL), a double anterior horn or flipped meniscus (anterior fragment displacement), and a disproportionally small posterior horn (the end or the beginning of the longitudinal tear) (Fig. 3). It is relevant suspecting this lesion of the LM if it appears as a fragment located just posterior to the ACL. Mimics of the double PCL sign include a prominent ligament of Humphrey, a meniscomeniscal ligament, and intercondylar osseous bodies (vv 3).

BLOKS

The BLOKS is based on both subregional cartilage score and cartilage integrity score. The knee surfaces are subdivided in different zones (patella medial/lateral, condyle medial/lateral,

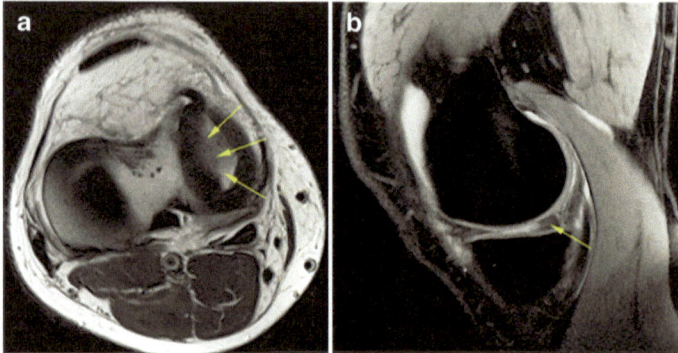

Figure 3 Meniscal bucket-handle tear: axial TSE T2-weighted image (**a**) shows the displacement of the meniscal "handle" (*arrows*); note that the inner rim and the meniscus have a different shape and dimension: this is may be helpful for distinguish a meniscal flap lesion (same dimension of the upper and lower valves of the meniscus) from a bucket handle tear (inner portion displaced from a longitudinal/parallel lesion to the C-shaped fibers of the meniscus); on (**b**) sagittal DESS FS image, an absent body meniscus may be seen and horizontal complex tear is present (*arrow*)

tibial plateau medial/lateral, intercondylar zone, and tibial spines). The first score is assigned based on the size of the cartilage damage related to each zone: 0 no cartilage loss, 1 for <10 % of the zone, 2 for 10–75 % of the zone, and 3 for >75 % of the zone of cartilage layer area. The second score evaluates the percentage of full-thickness cartilage damage in the zone: 0 for no significant cartilage loss, 1 for <10 % of the zone, 2 for 10–75 % of the zone, and 3 for >75 % of the zone.

Suggested Reading

Ahn JH, Kim KI, Wang JH et al (2015) Arthroscopic repair of bucket-handle tears of the lateral meniscus. Knee Surg Sports Traumatol Arthrosc 23(1):205–210

Gudbergsen H, Lohmander LS, Jones G et al (2013) Correlations between radiographic assessments and MRI features of knee osteoarthritis – a cross-sectional study. Osteoarthritis Cartilage 21(4):535–543

Hunter DJ, Lo GH, Gale D, Grainger AJ et al (2008) The reliability of a new scoring system for knee osteoarthritis MRI and the validity of bone marrow lesion assessment: BLOKS (Boston Leeds Osteoarthritis Knee Score). Ann Rheum Dis 67(2):206–211. Epub 2007 May 1. Review

Nguyen JC, De Smet AA, Graf BK et al (2014) MR imaging-based diagnosis and classification of meniscal tears. Radiographics 34(4):981–999

Prasad A, Brar R, Rana S (2014) MRI imaging of displaced meniscal tears: report of a case highlighting new potential pitfalls of the MRI signs. Indian J Radiol Imaging 24(3):291–296

Türkmen F, Korucu IH, Sever C et al (2014) Free medial meniscal fragment which mimics the dislocated bucket-handle tear on MRI. Case Rep Orthop 2014:647491

Van der Esch M, Knoop J, Hunter DJ, Klein JP et al (2013) The association between reduced knee joint proprioception and medial meniscal abnormalities using MRI in knee osteoarthritis: results from the Amsterdam osteoarthritis cohort. Osteoarthritis Cartilage 21(5):676–681

C

Cartilage, Compositional MR Imaging

With the compositional cartilage imaging, an advanced MR tool, it is possible to detect biochemical changes that antici- pate morphological cartilage interruption. Each compositional technique is based on the characterization of macromolecular content and organization of the chondral layer. In particular, two aspects are mainly considered: first, the collagen fiber network of the extracellular matrix, extremely arranged in the space for its tensile and shear straight properties, and, second, matrix content of GAGs that is negatively charged due to the presence of carboxyl and sulfate groups. Most validated techniques are the following:

- *T2 mapping*: T2 mapping is based on the differences in T2 times of dissimilar zones and organization of the collagen matrix. Ordinarily with MR imaging, when a good contrast between fluid and cartilage is present, it is possible to give a subjective assessment of cartilage T2 changes, whereas T2 mapping provides numerical data by creating a color scale map representing the variations in relaxation time within cartilage. The areas with higher T2 than that of normal carti- lage represent zones of early disruption and degeneration.

M. Osimani, C. Chillemi, *Knee Imaging*, A-Z Notes in Radiological   19
Practice and Reporting, DOI 10.1007/978-88-470-3950-6_3,
© Springer-Verlag Italia 2017

Another application of T2 maps could be the assessment of the achievement of cartilage repair.

- *dGEMRIC*: The dGEMRIC technique is based on the interaction between Gd-DTPA^{2-} and negatively charged GAGs. After the intravenous administration of Gd, this is more concentrated in areas with little content of GAGs, and this is observable on a T1-colored map, allowing a quantitative evaluation of GAGs. After administration of Gd, the joint is moved for at least 15 min, to allow the infiltration of the Gd in the chondral clefts.

- *T1ρ*: T1ρ measures the interactions between motion-constrained water molecules and their local macromolecular environment, so this technique may provide an ideal measure of cartilage composition in collagen and GAGs and a depletion of those may result in higher T1ρ values than normal cartilage, especially in the first stage of OA. However, T1ρ measure is not specific for GAGs depletion, and a higher T1ρ may imply other macromolecules reducing or collagen fiber "mal-orientation." Although this technique is disposable as add-on pack in most MRI scanners and several studies tested its performance in the early stage of the OA, there are few studies about the performance of the technique in the evaluation of chondral implant and repair, and this is the theoretically ideal field of employment (low specificity with highest sensitivity).

- *Sodium imaging*: On the basis of mentioned negative charge of GAGs, sodium occurs naturally in the cartilage matrix as positive ion. This promising technique may hypothetically map the depletion of GAGs but is actually limited by the requirement of special hardware and low SNR of the images obtained.

- *Diffusion-weighted imaging*: The diffusion of water is higher in cartilage when the strict organization of collagen fibers is intact; an increase in ADC, although with low quality images, may represent a first stage of chondral layer disruption, but, at the date of this publication, further studies are necessary to improve the acquisition parameters and technique.

Cartilage, Semiquantitative Morphologic Assessment

Chondral defects and bone remodeling during OA process must be assessed in clinical routine using Outerbridge grading system, but in some patients, especially young athletes, or in studies in which the postoperative success has to be estimated before and after surgery, the use of semiquantitative scoring methods such as those known as WORMS, BLOKS, and MOAKS (see lemmas) must be assessed. Such scoring systems are based on the evaluation of chondral deficiency in conjunction with those of the menisci, subchondral bone, and synovial inflammation.

MRI Techniques and Sequences

For the correct assessment of those scores, it is crucial to pay attention on the imaging protocol used; an optimal contrast between the cartilage and articular fluid and a fine BML estimation and meniscal lesions must be evaluated by dedicated protocols including two- or three-dimensional techniques. The basic protocol provides at least a PD or intermediate-weighted FS sequences in all planes plus one non-FS T1 weighted (coronal preferred). These sequences enable to find also loose bodies and to assess the quality of subchondral bone (granulation tissue vs. sclerosis). If 3D technique were available, a GRE or SSFP must be included. When a chondral defect is suspected on images acquired on low-field articular-dedicated scanner (<0.7 Tesla), we suggest to repeat the exam on a high-field scanner (≥1.5 Tesla), because of the lack of correct contrast between the cartilage and fluid with low-field magnets, which may cause false-positive results. The following are the dedicated sequences for cartilage evaluation:

- *Fat saturation techniques*: These are commonly used but time consuming and sensitive to motion artifacts. It may be replaced by volumetric gradient-recalled echo techniques.
- *2D PD or FS TSE*: This is generally used in the clinical routine. The use of intermediate echo times of 30–60 ms may be helpful, in order to avoid magic-angle artifact and to obtain more contrast between cartilage and articular fluid. Partial volume effects must be considered because of anisotropic acquisition.
- *3D FSE*: This is recently introduced to outperform 2D techniques limits. 3D FSE imaging permits to perform high-quality multiplanar reformations for cartilage segmentation and to evaluate menisci, ligaments, and subchondral damages. An example of 3D FSE is the SPACE (Siemens vendor)/CUBE (GE vendor)/VISTA (Philips vendor) acquisition method, that is, a long acquisition technique with poor cartilage-to-fluid contrast.
- *3D SPGR*: This is the ideal acquisition technique for the assessment of cartilage morphology, especially when a segmentation is required. The sequence may be performed when a long acquisition time is possible (sensitivity to susceptibility artifacts) and during the acute phase of a traumatic chondral lesion when articular fluid is copious (contrast between cartilage and fluid).
- *3D DESS*: This is similar to SPGR but more time efficient with higher SNR and higher chondral contrast (Fig. 1).
- *3D VIPR SSFP*: This sequence outperforms the limits of the GRE imaging with a good contrast between fluid and cartilage. The VIPR 3D radial acquisition of the k-space assents both to reduce the acquisition time and to assess cartilage, menisci, and BMLs, with good accuracy also in bone edema (Fig. 2).

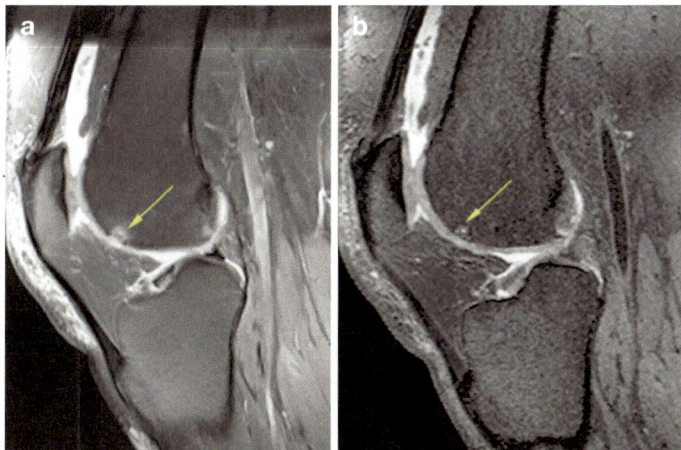

FIGURE 1 Osteochondral lesion: sagittal PD FS (**a**) and DESS (**b**) show an osteochondral lesion on the anterior aspect of the femoral condyle. Note that on DESS image it is possible to identify granulation tissue on the defect and sclerotic margin; in PD image the bone edema did not permit a correct staging and description of the lesion (*arrows* in **a** and **b**)

Chondrocalcinosis

Similar to a meniscal ossicle, chondrocalcinosis represents a diffuse calcification of meniscal matrix and can result in increased meniscal signal intensity, thus decreasing the accuracy of MR imaging for detection of tears. Otherwise by the alteration described in the previous lemma, radiographs reduce misdiagnosis. Prevalence increases with age.

Collateral Ligaments, Tear

Lesions of medial collateral ligament (MCL) and lateral collateral ligament (LCL) are very frequent because of their association

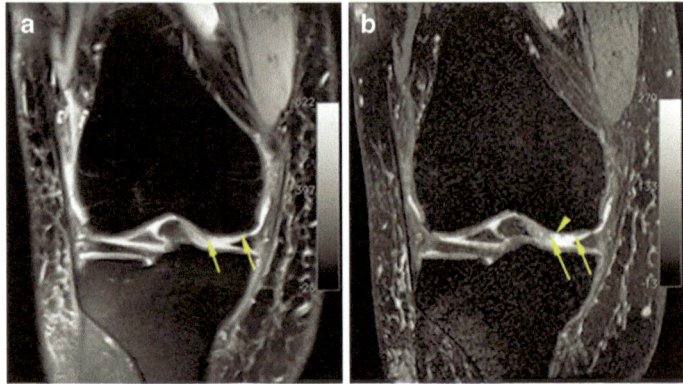

FIGURE 2 Osteochondral lesion: coronal PD FS (**a**) and true-FISP (**b**) show an osteochondral lesion on the articular side of the medial femoral condyle (*arrows* on **a** and **b**). Note that on true-FISP image, it is possible to assess residual cartilage covering the subchondral bone; in PD image the bone edema did not permit a correct staging and description of the lesion (*arrowhead* in **b**)

in meniscal or cruciate ligaments tears (e.g., O'Donoghue's unhappy triad). The medial injury is the most common ligamentous injury of the knee, as the prevalence of sport-related valgus stress on the knee and the complex three anatomic layers of the medial capsule (see MCL, anatomy lemma). Tears of LCL are also very often associated with ALC or PCL lesions, because of the stabilization function of the posterolateral corner.

- *Radiography*: Plain film may demonstrate associated bone lesions as calcifications in the chronic phase of the tear as calcification of MCL, named Pellegrini-Stieda disease or avulsion fractures as Segond fracture or fracture of the fibular head in the LCL lesions.
- *Computed tomography*: This has similar findings of the plain film and is helpful in doubtful cases.
- *Ultrasounds*: Ultrasonography may be a help as a "screening" exam because of its high accuracy in MCL tears

detection. A MCL partial tear appears as hypoechoic ligament with fluid surrounding the superficial or both deep
layers. Ligament disruption appears as discontinuity of the
fibers. It is also useful to integrate the exam to anterior and
posterior layers of the capsule as a MCL tear often involves
the oblique ligament or the patellar retinacula. In this manner, parameniscal cysts or intramuscular hematoma of vastus medialis may be found as associated lesions. Stress
scansions of both knees may evidence an enlargement of
medial articular rim as expression of biomechanical failure of the fibers.

- *Magnetic resonance*: To diagnose collateral ligament tears
  is crucial in the assessment of Coronal images. Fluid-
  sensitive sequences, such as PD fat suppressed, detect
  edema surrounding the ligaments, and T1-weighted images
  are helpful for the anatomical assessment of fibers integrity. Lesions located mainly in the posterior lateral or
  medial corner of the capsules are detectable easily through
  axial images. A grading system of tears is traditionally
  used both for medial and lateral ligament. In grade I, intact
  fibers are revealed (microscopic lesion) with surrounding
  edema, seen better in PD FS coronal images. The ligament
  must be closely near the femoral and tibial bones and
  stretched (above all MCL). We confirm this feature also in
  contiguous axial images avoiding potential pitfalls related
  to incorrect orientation of coronal images on axial and sagittal planes. In grade II, surrounding edema is more evident, also as intermediate signal in T1-weighted images
  and areas of intermediate signal appears also among the
  fibers. In this grade the ligament (MCL or LCL) have a
  partial tear. In grade III the retraction of fibers is due to
  total lesion of the ligament, and the resulting instability is
  more evident, also for meniscal or cruciate-associated
  tears. Bone edema occurs when ligament tear causes a
  periostal stripping near the insertion (femoral or tibial).

In the chronic phase of a lesion of the MCL, the ligament appears thickened and with low signal (approximately 12 months). An abnormal healing process is represented by the calcification of the MCL, best appreciated on radiographs (see Pellegrini-Stieda) (Fig. 3).

- In the evaluation of LCL tears, we must take into mind some differences such as the ligament visualization in consecutive coronal images (the ligament course is posterior-oblique; see anatomy lemma) and less evident fluid surrounding the ligament in partial tears. Morphologic changes are the most specific sign with serpiginous, deflected, and discontinuous fibers (eventually bone avulsion of fibular head). As previously discussed, also LCL tears are very often associated with central-pivot ligaments lesions.

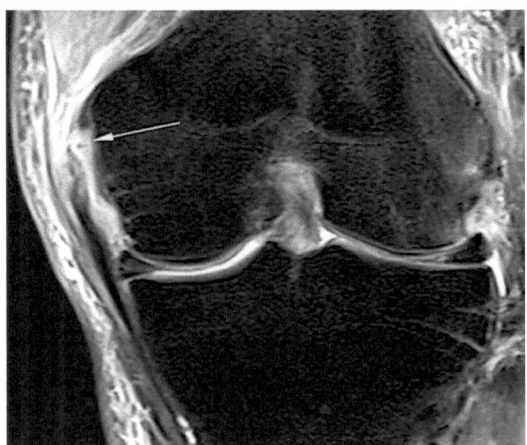

FIGURE 3 Grade III complete MCL lesion. The image shows complete lesion of the MCL with retraction of distal fibers. Note the communication between articular fluid and extra-articular tissues (*arrow*)

Coronary Ligaments

The coronary ligaments (meniscotibial ligaments) arise from the posterior horn of the LM to the tibial plateau. Together with meniscal root, this is a static stabilizer of the LM. The absence of the coronary ligaments and popliteomeniscal fascicles represents a specific MR sign of Wrisberg variant discoid meniscus (see lemma).

- *MRI*: The coronary ligaments are found along either side of the popliteal hiatus with the anterior band attachment generally easiest to identify several millimeters distal to the articular surface and best seen on posterior fat-suppressed proton density-weighted coronal. We can find also a fluid-filled recess.

Suggested Reading

Alizai H, Virayavanich W, Joseph GB et al (2014) Cartilage lesion score: comparison of a quantitative assessment score with established semi-quantitative MR scoring systems. Radiology 271(2):479–487

Choi JA, Gold GE (2011) MR imaging of articular cartilage physiology. Magn Reson Imaging Clin N Am 19(2):249–282. doi:10.1016/j.mric.2011.02.010. Review

Crema MD, Roemer FW, Marra MD et al (2011) Articular cartilage in the knee: current MR imaging techniques and applications in clinical practice and research. Radiographics 31(1):37–61

de Windt TS, Welsch GH, Brittberg M et al (2013) Is magnetic resonance imaging reliable in predicting clinical outcome after articular cartilage repair of the knee? A systematic review and meta-analysis. Am J Sports Med 41(7):1695–1702

Gallo MC, Wyatt C, Pedoia V, et al (2016) T1ρ and T2 relaxation times are associated with progression of hip osteoarthritis. Osteoarthritis Cartilage. pii: S1063-4584(16)01062-1

Jungmann PM, Baum T, Bauer JS et al (2014) Cartilage repair surgery: outcome evaluation by using noninvasive cartilage biomarkers based on quantitative MRI techniques? Biomed Res Int 2014:840170

Surowiec RK, Lucas EP, Ho CP (2014) Quantitative MRI in the evaluation of articular cartilage health: reproducibility and variability with a focus on T2 mapping. Knee Surg Sports Traumatol Arthrosc 22(6):1385–1395

Trattnig S, Millington SA, Szomolanyi P et al (2007) MR imaging of osteo-chondral grafts and autologous chondrocyte implantation. Eur Radiol 17(1):103–118. Epub 2006 Jun 27. Review

Zhong H, Miller DJ, Urish KL (2016) T2 map signal variation predicts symptomatic osteoarthritis progression: data from the Osteoarthritis Initiative. Skeletal Radiol 45(7):909–913

D

Deep Lateral Femoral Notch Sign

The deep lateral femoral notch sign, although uncommon, is subchondral fracture lines or cortical contour flattening appreciated in sagittal planes or lateral radiographs and is quite specific for ACL tear. It is caused by impact injury of the lateral femoral condylopatellar notch onto the tibia. A notch depth of over 1.5–2 mm is diagnostic.

Discoid Meniscus

Discoid meniscus is a normal anatomic variant that is seen in 0.8–3.0 % of knees, characterized by a wider than normal meniscal body that results in greater coverage of the tibia. It may lead to abnormal biomechanical forces across the knee. Watanabe and Takeda described three types of discoid menisci: incomplete, complete, and Wrisberg variant.

- MRI: In the incomplete variant, the discoid may be seen as meniscal body evidence on three consecutive 3–4 mm sections on sagittal plane (tibial coverage <80 % on axial plane),

M. Osimani, C. Chillemi, *Knee Imaging*, A-Z Notes in Radiological Practice and Reporting, DOI 10.1007/978-88-470-3950-6_4,
© Springer-Verlag Italia 2017

while in the complete, the body may be seen in all sections. These types represent the "stable" variants of LM (intact posterior meniscofemoral ligament). Wrisberg variant represents the unstable variant and lacks the normal posterior coronary ligament and capsular attachments (see specific lemma).

Distal Femur Fractures

Two main causes are recognized in distal femoral fractures: high-energy trauma in young population (<40 years; male predominance) and low-energy trauma in osteoporotic population (>50 years; female predominance). Identification of articular surface involvement, fragmentation, and deformation of metaphysis and epiphysis in distal femur fracture are crucial in terms of surgical and nonsurgical procedures. Osteoporotic fractures can be problematic for fixation. Soft tissue injuries can be associated as meniscal and ligaments tears; neurovascular injuries can also occur but rarely. Femur fractures may be classified on the basis of Müller classification, in which category A are the extra-articular fractures, category B are partial articular factures (part of the articular surface remains attached to the diaphysis), and category C are the complete articular fractures (both condyles separated from diaphysis). Every category is subdivided based on fracture direction, grade, and complexity of fragmentation.

- *Radiography*: X-ray is the standard evaluative technique for this type of fracture. It shows with high diagnostic accuracy on the fracture itself but is not appropriate in assessing the involvement of intra-articular fractures with a high frequency of false negatives. AP and lateral projection are sufficient for the standard identification of these fractures. Oblique view may support the standard analysis, but if the CT scanning is available, it can be avoided.
- *CT scan*: Once the fracture is identified by radiographs or if it has not been identified but clinically suspected, a CT scan

must be undertaken. Indeed, the factors that influence the fracture management include: the intra-articular involvement and the complexity of fragmentation and displacement. Everything can be evaluated by means of the CT scan with the use of MPR and VR reconstruction. It is also possible to evaluate indirect signs of possible vascular injuries such as soft tissues infarction seen as increased density or the presence of sharp displaced fragments near the vascular axis. In cases where limb perfusion is of concern, it is crucial that an angiography, perfusion CT, or Doppler exam is performed, keeping in mind that distal pulses do not exclude the presence of vascular injury.

- In cases where it is necessary to apply temporary external fixation devices, it is recommended to undertake the CT scan prior to positioning because of the artifacts derived by beam hardening.
- *MRI*: MR may be useful for the assessment of meniscal tears or capsular ligament injury. As in the CT scan, if there is need to use external devices and an MRI is recommended, it should be undertaken first.

Suggested Reading

Connolly JF (1989) Closed treatment of pelvic and lower extremity fractures. Clin Orthop Relat Res 240:115–128. Review

Lee SH, Baek JR, Han SB, Park SW (2005) Stress fractures of the femoral diaphysis in children: a report of 5 cases and review of literature. J Pediatr Orthop 25(6):734–738. Review

Mellado JM, Ramos A, Salvadó E et al (2002) Avulsion fractures and chronic avulsion injuries of the knee: role of MR imaging. Eur Radiol 12(10):2463–2473. Epub 2002 Mar 23. Review

Tyler W, Bukata S, O'Keefe R (2014) Atypical femur fractures. Clin Geriatr Med 30(2):349–359

Wehrli FW, Saha PK, Gomberg BR et al (2002) Role of magnetic resonance for assessing structure and function of trabecular bone. Top Magn Reson Imaging 13(5):335–355. Review

E

Extensor Mechanism

The extensor mechanism is a complex biomechanical system that prejudices quadriceps muscle group, the quadriceps tendon, the patella, the patellar tendon, and the insertion of the patellar tendon on the tibial tubercle. The extensor mechanism, mostly used to maintain the upright position, is based on the interaction between the activity of extensor muscles and passive stabilizers as the bone morphology and ligament integrity.

- *MRI*—we recommend focusing on at least two "key zones" on axial and sagittal T2-weighted MR images: (1) the geometry of the femoral-patellar joint, with femoral trochlea deep enough and lateral aspect high enough to ensure an anatomical "wall" during the movement track of the patella, and (2) the MFPL that avoids the patellar lateral displacement during the knee flexion. It is important to assess the elements of this medial capsular side into three laminar structures:

  - The surface layer composed of the fascia of the sartorius muscle.

M. Osimani, C. Chillemi, *Knee Imaging*, A-Z Notes in Radiological Practice and Reporting, DOI 10.1007/978-88-470-3950-6_5,
© Springer-Verlag Italia 2017

- – The intermediate layer formed by MFPL, similar to a fan, from the medial patella to the medial femoral condyle (together with the retinacula).
- – The inner layer represented by the knee capsule. On the basis of the correct evaluation of this two "key zones," we may assess both risk factors for patella-femoral instability (see lemmas Trochlear Dysplasia, Patella Alta, and TT-TG Distance) and MRI features after patellar displacement (see lemma).

Suggested Reading

Bonnin M, Lustig S, Huten D (2016) Extensor tendon ruptures after total knee arthroplasty. Orthop Traumatol Surg Res 102(Suppl 1):S21–S31

Merrow AC, Reiter MP, Zbojniewicz AM et al (2014) Avulsion fractures of the pediatric knee. Pediatr Radiol 44(11):1436–1445; quiz 1433-6

Yablon CM, Pai D, Dong Q et al (2014) Magnetic resonance imaging of the extensor mechanism. Magn Reson Imaging Clin N Am 22(4):601–620

F

Femorotibial Translation

Anterior translocation of the tibia is the mirror of ACL incompetency. This secondary sign must be sought on lateral radiographs or MRI sagittal planes with a perpendicular line from the lateral condyle to the posterior-lateral tibial plateau. If the tibia shifts anteriorly more than 5 mm, acute or chronic ACL tear is likely. An anterior tibial translation >7 mm is fully diagnostic of ACL tear.

Flap Tear

A flap tear is an evolution of a horizontal MM tear with superior (more common) or inferior displacement of the fragment (one of the two halves of the meniscus).

- *Fragment* may be displaced also inferior and medial to the tibial plateau, near to the MCL, and has to be noticed in the report as the arthroscopist may not display that fragment.

M. Osimani, C. Chillemi, *Knee Imaging*, A-Z Notes in Radiological   35
Practice and Reporting, DOI 10.1007/978-88-470-3950-6_6,
© Springer-Verlag Italia 2017

Suggested Reading

Alatakis S, Naidoo P (2009) MR imaging of meniscal and cartilage injuries of the knee. Magn Reson Imaging Clin N Am 17(4):741–756

Davis KW, Rosas HG, Graf BK (2013) Magnetic resonance imaging and arthroscopic appearance of the menisci of the knee. Clin Sports Med 32(3):449–475

G

Ghost Meniscus

Ghost meniscus is the absence of half bow tie when a full-thickness radial tear involves the entire meniscus. This results in a no in-plane residual normal meniscus on MR images. If this sign is suspected, it has to be confirmed on another scan plane (cleft plus ghost) (Figs. 1 and 2).

M. Osimani, C. Chillemi, *Knee Imaging*, A-Z Notes in Radiological Practice and Reporting, DOI 10.1007/978-88-470-3950-6_7,
© Springer-Verlag Italia 2017

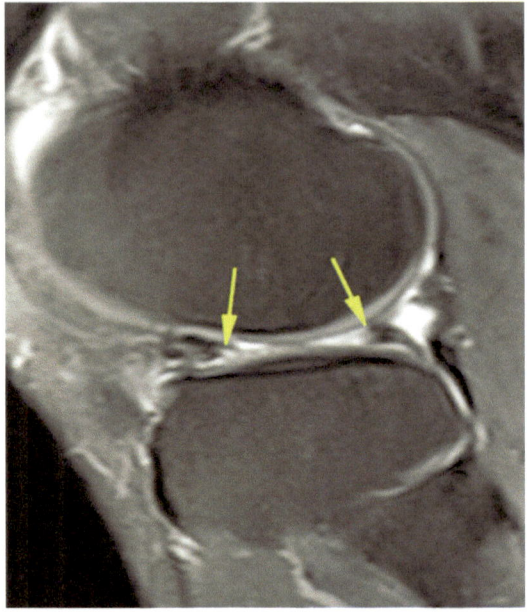

FIGURE 1 Large ghost meniscus: note the absent bow-tie sign (*arrows*). A longitudinal lesion of lateral meniscus should be suspected

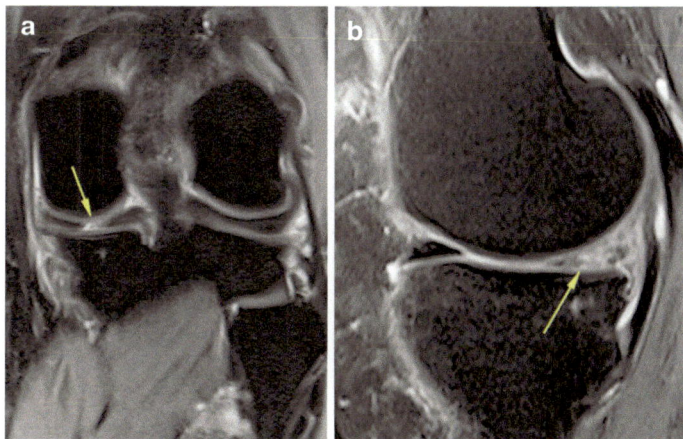

FIGURE 2 Radial lesion signs: the image shows a radial lesion of the posterior horn of the medial meniscus (*arrows* in **a** and **b**). Note the "cleft" sign in (**a**) coronal image (see lemma) and typical "ghost meniscus" in (**b**) sagittal corresponding image

Suggested Reading

Papalia R, Vasta S, Franceschi F et al (2013) Meniscal root tears: from basic science to ultimate surgery. Br Med Bull 106:91–115

H

Hypermobile Lateral Meniscus

Hypermobile lateral meniscus (or flipped meniscus) has the same absence of posterior horn coronary and popliteomeniscal ligaments of the Wrisberg variant of discoid meniscus, but with an absence of discoid body morphology. The symptoms range from asymptomatic patients to pain related to continuous subluxation (above all in forced flexion).

- *MRI*: at the beginning, most of the MR exams of patients with a hypermobile lateral meniscus are interpreted as negative. This depends on the compliance of the radiologist in searching these thin structures and above all to image quality. Some authors suggested the execution of a parasagittal plane parallel to the popliteal course. In our opinion this is poorly reasonable because of the condition that is generally suspected after a strong image review, often by indirect sign as a meniscal flounce or radial lesion of the anterior horn or body of LM (subluxation expects). In our experience when we find an excessive fluid between popliteus tendon and posterior horn of lateral meniscus, it is reasonable to check the posterior capsule integrity (a thin fluid collection among the popliteus tendon is however normal).

M. Osimani, C. Chillemi, *Knee Imaging*, A-Z Notes in Radiological
Practice and Reporting, DOI 10.1007/978-88-470-3950-6_8,
© Springer-Verlag Italia 2017

Suggested Reading

Moser MW, Dugas J, Hartzell J et al (2007) A hypermobile Wrisberg variant lateral discoid meniscus seen on MRI. Clin Orthop Relat Res 456:264–267

Van Steyn MO, Mariscalco MW, Pedroza AD et al (2014) The hypermobile lateral meniscus: a retrospective review of presentation, imaging, treatment, and results. Knee Surg Sports Traumatol Arthrosc 24(5):1555–1559

I

Iliotibial Tract or Band

This is common fascia of the tensor of fasciae latae, gluteus maximus, and medius. Its distal insertion is on the tibial Gerdy tubercle and proximal to the knee; it inserts on the supracondylar tubercle of the lateral femoral condyle with the intermuscular septum.

With functional flexion and extension of the knee, the iliotibial band passes over the lateral femoral epicondyle with an inflammatory response in the soft tissues.

On MRI the tissues around the iliotibial band become hyperintense on T2-weighted images, with cystic organization in the late or chronic phase of the inflammation. On axial images the iliotibial band inflammation has to be differentiated by the normal lateral recess, as the recess is located anterior to the femoral epicondyle, while the iliotibial band and the collection fluid are located posteriorly.

M. Osimani, C. Chillemi, *Knee Imaging*, A-Z Notes in Radiological
Practice and Reporting, DOI 10.1007/978-88-470-3950-6_9,
© Springer-Verlag Italia 2017

Iliotibial Band Avulsion Fracture

This fracture involves the anterolateral corner of the tibia, known as Gerdy tubercle in pure varus force. Rarely seen as an isolated injury because varus stress happens usually with flexed knee; other stabilizer injuries had to be evaluated as well as ACL disruption.

- *MRI*: MRI is the method of choice revealing avulsion and retraction of the iliotibial band from its distal insertion on the Gerdy tubercle.

Suggested Reading

Bencardino JT, Rosenberg ZS, Brown RR et al (2000) Traumatic musculo-tendinous injuries of the knee: diagnosis with MR imaging. Radiographics 20 Spec No:S103–S120. Review

Fairclough J, Hayashi K, Toumi H et al (2006) The functional anatomy of the iliotibial band during flexion and extension of the knee: implications for understanding iliotibial band syndrome. J Anat 208(3):309–316

Fairclough J, Hayashi K, Toumi H et al (2007) Is iliotibial band syndrome really a friction syndrome? J Sci Med Sport 10(2):74–76; discussion 77–78

J

No lemma

M. Osimani, C. Chillemi, *Knee Imaging*, A-Z Notes in Radiological
Practice and Reporting, DOI 10.1007/978-88-470-3950-6_10,
© Springer-Verlag Italia 2017

K

Kellgren and Lawrence System

Classification for grading knee osteoarthritis. Signs must be observed on weight-bearing AP radiographs and otherwise from Ahlback classification; the grading is more centered on bone remodeling. According to the system, we can find four grades of severity: (0) absence of radiographic signs of osteoarthritis; (1) initial osteophytosis; (2) definite osteophytes and narrowing of joint rim space; (3) well appreciable multiple osteophytosis, sclerosis, and initial bone remodeling; and (4) joint rim not appreciable with severe sclerosis and bone remodeling.

Knee MRI Study, Protocol

• Standard/routine exam (scan plane, sequence, weighing, TR, TE, matrix/nex, thickness mm/gap, Fov cm, others):

  – CORONAL, SE, T1, 690, 14, 512/2, 4/0, 4, 14
  – CORONAL, DESS, DE, 24, 7, 256/2, 1/20 %, 14

M. Osimani, C. Chillemi, *Knee Imaging*, A-Z Notes in Radiological Practice and Reporting, DOI 10.1007/978-88-470-3950-6_11, © Springer-Verlag Italia 2017

- SAGITTAL, TSE-PD, PD, 2500, 26, 512/2, 4/0, 4, 14
- SAGITTAL, SE, T1, 690, 14, 512/2, 4/0, 4, 14
- AXIAL, TSE-PD, PD, 4000, 26, 256/2, 4/0, 4, 14, FS

• Postoperative meniscus add-on sequences (scan plane, sequence, weighing, TR, TE, matrix/nex, thickness mm/gap, Fov cm, others):

- SAGITTAL, TSE-PD, PD, 4000, 26, 256/2, 4/0, 4, 14, FS

• Postoperative ACL add-on sequences (scan plane, sequence, weighing, TR, TE, matrix/nex, thickness mm/gap, Fov cm, others):

- AXIAL, TSE, T2, 3550, 30, 512/2, 4/0, 4, 14
- SAGITTAL, TSE, T2, 4000, 102, 512/2, 4/0, 4, 14

• Postoperative knee Gd add-on sequences (scan plane, sequence, weighing, TR, TE, matrix/nex, thickness mm/gap, Fov cm, others):

- SAGITTAL-AXIAL, SE, T1, 589, 14, 512/2, 4/0, 4, 14, FS

Knee Radiographic Projection, AP Knee

Rationale: shows femorotibial articulation

• *Technique:* patient in supine. Cassette under the knee with femoral condyles parallel to the grid. Beam direction: anteroposterior perpendicular to the grid, level 1–2 cm distal to the patella
• *Key points:* distal femur and tibial plateau fractures

Knee Radiographic Projection, Camp Coventry PA Axial Projection-Tunnel View

Rationale: shows posterior aspect of femoral condyles, the intercondylar tibial spines, and the intercondylar notch

- *Technique:* patient in prone with the knee in 40° of flexion. Cassette under the knee. Beam direction: posteroanterior cranio-caudal with an angle of 40° from the vertical plane
- *Key points:* to assess distal femur fracture

Knee Radiographic Projection, Cross Table Lateral View

Rationale: shows the femorotibial and patellofemoral articulation

- *Technique:* patient in supine decubitus with the uninjured leg raised and the injured one extended. Grid lateral to the affected knee. Beam direction: horizontal
- *Key points:* to assess tibial plateau, distal femur, and patellar fractures

Knee Radiographic Projection, Knee Sunrise View

Rationale: shows the patellofemoral articulation (tangential aspect of the patella)

- *Technique:* patient in prone with the knee in 115° of flexion (angle of flexion open distally). Cassette under the knee. Beam direction: posteroanterior cranio-caudal with an angle of 40° from the vertical plane
- *Key points:* to assess patellar fractures

Knee Radiographic Projection, Lateral Knee

Rationale: shows the femorotibial and patellofemoral articulation

- *Technique:* patient in lateral decubitus of the affected side knee with 30° of flexion. Grid under the knee. Beam direction: above the knee with caudal-cranial inclination of 5°
- *Key points:* to assess tibial plateau, distal femur, and patellar fractures

Knee Radiographic Projection, Merchant Bilateral Tangential Skyline Projection

Rationale: shows the patellofemoral articulation

- *Technique:* patient in supine with the knee in 45 of flexion at the table edge. Cassette held perpendicular to the tibia. *Beam direction:* cranio-caudal direct to the patella with 60° from vertical plane or 30° from horizontal plane
- *Key points:* to assess patellar fractures

Knee Radiographic Projection, Rosenberg

Rationale: shows the femorotibial articulation; it is recommended when an articular fracture is suspected on the medial sides of the condyles.

- *Technique:* weight bearing with the knee in 45° of flexion. Grid anterior to the knee. Beam direction: posteroanterior with an inclination of 10° caudal from the horizontal plane
- *Key points:* to assess tibial plateau and distal femur fractures

Suggested Reading

Berkes MB, Little MT, Pardee NC et al (2013) Defining the lateral and accessory views of the patella: an anatomic and radiographic study with implications for fracture treatment. J Orthop Trauma 27(12):663–671

Heng HY, Bin Abd Razak HR, Mitra AK (2015) Radiographic grading of the patellofemoral joint is more accurate in skyline compared to lateral views. Ann Transl Med 3(18):263

Kalinosky B, Sabol JM, Piacsek K et al (2011) Quantifying the tibiofemoral joint space using x-ray tomosynthesis. Med Phys 38(12):6672–6682

Koike M, Nose H, Takagi S et al (2015) A skyline-view imaging technique for axial projection of the patella: a clinical study. Radiol Phys Technol 8(2):174–177

Weber E, Theisen D, Wilmes P et al (2016) A new quantitative measure for radiologic osteoarthritis of the lateral knee compartment distinguishes patients with longstanding lateral meniscectomy from non-pathological knees. Knee Surg Sports Traumatol Arthrosc 24(5):1569–1574

L

Lateral Knee Capsule

The later capsule has several ligamentous and tendon structures divisible in anterior stabilizers and posterior ones. In the anterior side, we find the iliotibial tract (see lemma) and the superior and inferior retinacula with the vastus lateralis muscle. The posterior-lateral side was considered as distinct functional tendon-ligamentous unit, known as "arcuate ligament complex" (see lemma).

Suggested Reading

Bolog N, Hodler J (2007) MR imaging of the posterolateral corner of the knee. Skeletal Radiol 36(8):715–728, Epub 2007 Mar 2. Review

Jia Y, Gou W, Geng L et al (2012) Anatomic proximity of the peroneal nerve to the posterolateral corner of the knee determined by MR imaging. Knee 19(6):766–768

Peduto AJ, Nguyen A, Trudell DJ et al (2008) Popliteomeniscal fascicles: anatomic considerations using MR arthrography in cadavers. AJR Am J Roentgenol 190(2):442–448

M. Osimani, C. Chillemi, *Knee Imaging*, A-Z Notes in Radiological   53
Practice and Reporting, DOI 10.1007/978-88-470-3950-6_12,
© Springer-Verlag Italia 2017

M

Medial Knee Capsule

The medial region of the knee capsule has three static main stabilizers: the superficial MCL, the deep MCL, and the posterior oblique ligament. According to Warren and Marshall, the capsule may be divided into a three-layer structure with the superficial MCL as the second layer between superficial sartorial fascia and the deep MCL.

The posterior portion of the ligament has a band of oblique fibers or posterior oblique ligament (see lemma), that develops the second and the third layers of the posteromedial capsule.

Menisci, Anatomy

Menisci are wedge-shaped, semilunar, fibrocartilaginous structures; there are two for the knee: medial meniscus (MM) and lateral meniscus (LM). Each meniscus can be subdivided into the anterior horn, body, posterior horn, and roots; furthermore, it is structured with a superior concave surface and a flat base

M. Osimani, C. Chillemi, *Knee Imaging*, A-Z Notes in Radiological
Practice and Reporting, DOI 10.1007/978-88-470-3950-6_13,
© Springer-Verlag Italia 2017

that attaches to the tibia. They also have a thicker peripheral portion and a thinner central free edge. LM and MM differ in some anatomical and functional characteristics; in fact MM is less mobile than LM (attached to PMC) and has a more open C-shaped pattern.

- *MRI*: At MR imaging, the menisci appear as low signal intensity structures related to a lack of mobile protons in the fibrocartilage and dephasing of hydrogen nuclei that results in shortening T2. On sagittal scans, they appear with a "bowtie" configuration, while they appear with a triangular or wedge shaped on coronal images.

  - Meniscal tears are characterizable with more accuracy with PD-weighted images instead of T1-weighted images. Therefore, short TE is significant when PD-weighted imaging is performed (less than 30 ms). For enough sections of menisci in the sagittal plane, a TR between 2000 and 3000 ms is suggested. GRE sequences are as correct as spin echo images for meniscal tears but inadequate to assess other knee structures.
  - Usually, images are performed with an extremity coil with high spatial resolution, a FOV of 15 cm or less, a preferred thickness of 3–4 mm, and a matrix of at least 192×256. Using a surface coil is also possible to obtain high-resolution images, with a smaller FOV and higher matrix values (displayed at 512×512).
  - With low field magnets (<1 Tesla), the use of "meniscal window" could help in the reviewing phase. This is obtained with a ROI centered on the meniscus, zoomed to 1.5–2X with a window width of 100–150 and level 1000.

Meniscal Cleft

The cleft sign is a not specific one; in fact it can be appreciated in both longitudinal and radial tears, depending on the location of it relative to the imaging plane. If the cleft is within the body, observed on coronal MR images, it is the result of a longitudinal tear. Instead if the cleft is within the horn, it is the result of a radial tear. The opposite combination holds true on sagittal MR images.

Meniscal Contusion

Meniscal contusion appears as diffuse internal increased signal that mimics a tear. A possible reason for the altered signal is to be referred to blood products that infiltrate along the meniscal fibers after compressive injury to the vascular zone. This is the consequence of a meniscal entrapment between the tibia and femur, often after an articular sprain, more frequently on LM as a result of a pivot shift. It is important to notice an indistinct and diffuse signal in contact with an articular surface to avoid misdiagnoses. Moreover, a high specific indirect sign is the presence of an adjacent bone contusion.

Meniscal, Degenerative Tear

Degenerative tears generally have a composite pattern and are more frequent in the posterior horn and mid-body of MM. Degenerative meniscus causes symptoms because of its

intrinsic innervations, which are most represented on the periphery and the anterior and posterior horns. Healing of the meniscus
is very uncertain because of poor vascularization of the periphery of the horns. In addition, chondral lesions cause a biochemical damage that adds to the mechanics overload and concur to
articular inflammation and instability.

- MRI signal changes are graded from I to III. In grade I, signal
  changes are globular and do not traverse the articular surface;
  in grade II, the signal becomes linear and does not involve the
  articular surface. These findings are compatible with intrasubstance degeneration in adults, while misdiagnosis has to be
  avoided in children as it is correlated with normal meniscus
  vascularity. In grade III, higher signal involves the superior or
  inferior articular surface, or both, and represent a true tear.

In patients with grade III degenerative tear, the treatment
must always be chosen upon the clinical and symptoms appearance, and not by imaging alone. Thus, mentioning a meniscal
degenerative tear in the report, without clinical symptoms correlation, should not induce the surgeon to proceed with
arthroscopy.

Meniscal Extrusion

Extrusion is present when the peripheral margin of the meniscus
extends 3 mm or more beyond the edge of the tibial plateau
because of loss of the meniscal hoop strength from tear of the
circumferentially oriented collagen bundles. About 76% of
medial root tears have extrusion, and 39% of extrusions have
medial root tears and can also be seen with complex tears, large
radial tears, and severe meniscal degeneration. The direction of
meniscal extrusion should be external on the capsule or on the
articular side.

- If this feature is noticed, it should be noteworthy to mention in the report because this is an indirect sign of an "unstable tear" (Fig. 1).

Meniscal Flounce

In a population with asymptomatic knees, 0.2–0.3 % of them could show at the arthroscopy a common sign with a wave

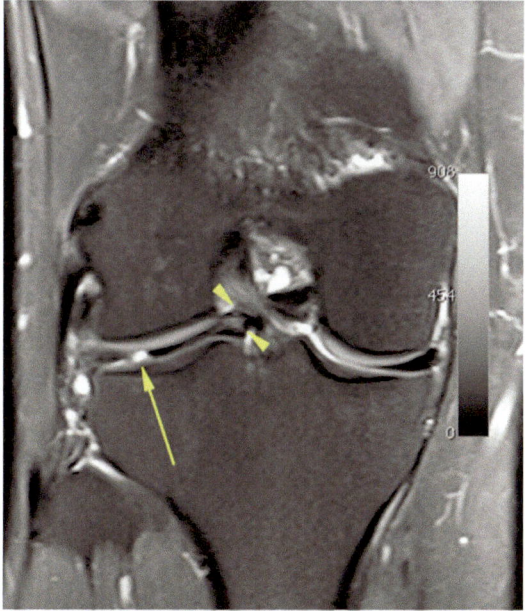

FIGURE 1 Meniscal extrusion: coronal PD FS image shows radial lesion (*arrow*) with extrusion of the lateral meniscus on the articular side (*arrowheads*). Note that the ACL represents a wall to meniscal displacement on the intercondilar notch

appearance of the free edge of the MM. This deformation is not a sign of tear. On coronal images, it may appear as truncated meniscus and mimic a radial tear (see lemma).

Meniscal Fraying

At arthroscopy, "fraying" is defined as surface irregularity along the meniscal free edge without an evident tear. At MR imaging, the free edge may appear with a loss of its sharp conical central edge; moreover, the posterior root ligaments may manifest thinner than usual, ill defined, and horizontally oriented with an increase of intrameniscal signal intensity contacting the articular surface. In our experience, improved in-plane resolution and thinner sections have resulted in MR imaging depiction of areas of meniscal fraying, which can involve the free edge of the body, the posterior horn, or the posterior root ligaments. However, doubtful cases still remain especially as regards LM instead of MM.

Meniscal Marching Cleft

If a radial tear is placed at the junction of the horn and body (obliquely oriented relative to both coronal and sagittal planes), it would appear as a "marching cleft" that progresses away from the free edge on contiguous MR imaging sections.

Meniscal Ossicle

Another case of misdiagnosed tear is meniscal ossicles due to an ossification focus of the posterior horn of the MM because of uncommon development, degeneration, or trauma. In fact on radiographs, the ossicle can be mistaken for a loose body, while at MR imaging, because of its increased signal intensity, it can mimic a tear (false-positive diagnosis). See also Chondrocalcinosis.

Meniscal Tear

Meniscal tears frequency raise with age, as part of a degenerative joint disease. Tears are more common in the posterior horn of the MM because, as described before, it has poor movement options; however, after injury in younger patients, meniscal tear is more common on LM. Regarding tears in the anterior horn, they are very uncommon to find isolated, accounting for 2 % and 16 % of MM and LM tears, respectively. In the presence of ACL tears, there is an increased prevalence of peripheral tears and a decreased sensitivity for detection of LM tears at MR imaging.

- *MRI*: On MR images, tears are recognized on the basis of meniscal morphology distortion or abnormal meniscal shape and an internal fissure with increased signal intensity (see imaging protocol under Menisci, anatomy) *clearly* contacting the articular surface (tibial or femoral). This finding has to be recognized at least on two or more images with "two-slice-touch" or/and "two-plane-touch" (sagittal plus coronal or sagittal plus axial). Increased intrasubstance signal intensity without extension to the articular surface is often not associated with a tear at surgery, and the PPV for a tear is 43 % in the MM and 18 % in the LM (best reported as a possible tear). Globular or linear increased intrameniscal signal intensity can be seen in normal meniscus vascularity in children, in adults with internal myxoid deterioration, and after trauma due to meniscal bruise.

- The higher meniscal signal of the tear is probably due to an increase in the "local spin density" and not from an increase in the T2 signal related to the loss of the normal collagen spiral, with a consequent increase of mobility of water molecules.
- Tears well seen on PD images should not be evident at T2-weighted images, unless there is a wide communication of the tear with joint fluid. If this signifying feature is observed, it should be mentioned in the report because this is an indirect sign of an "unstable tear."

- *Classification*: Although currently there is no clear tear classification system, it would be helpful to describe the morphology and the extension of the high signal fissure in the report. The most common tear patterns described are horizontal, longitudinal, radial, root, complex, displaced, and bucket-handle tears. Accurate description of tear morphology is decisive for treatment planning (conservative therapy, surgical repair, or partial or complete meniscectomy). Longitudinal tears are often repaired, whereas horizontal and radial tears may require surgery.

  - MR report about a meniscal tear should describe and characterize tear location, plane, shape, completeness, length, and number of tears.

- *Diagnostic errors*: False-positive errors may be experienced in the posterior horn of LM due to tears which are mistaken for normal anatomic structures or arterial pulsation or magic-angle effect that obscures a tear (fibers oriented 55° relative to the magnetic field). This effect commonly occurs within the posterior horn of LM and appears as increased signal intensity that does not extend to the meniscal surface, particularly on non-fluid-sensitive PD-weighted MR images.

Meniscal Tear, Displaced

A simple horizontal, longitudinal, or radial tear may progress and become displaced with the presence of free fragments, displaced flap tears, and bucket-handle tears (see lemma). A mechanical lock may be the effect of these tears and require surgery. An accurate description of fragment localization on report is essential to avoid missing small free fragments during arthroscopy. Flap tears occur six to seven times more frequently in the MM, where in two-thirds of cases, fragments are displaced posteriorly (near or posterior to the PCL); in the remaining cases, fragments displace into either the intercondylar notch or superior recess. Regarding LM, fragments are equally distributed along the posterior joint line and lateral recess.

Meniscal Tear, Horizontal

These tears usually occur in patients older than 40 years without trauma and are more common in the degenerative joint disease. The typical MR imaging appearance is a horizontally oblique-oriented line of high signal intensity parallel to the tibial plateau with contact of the articular surfaces or the central free edge; the tear dividing the meniscus into superior and inferior halves (Fig. 2). A direct communication with the joint fluid may appear

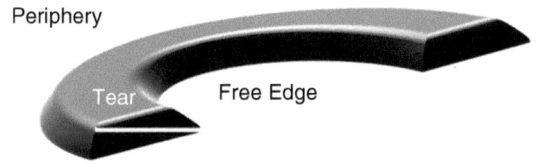

FIGURE 2 The scheme represents a horizontal tear. Take attention on the tear which divides the meniscus in two halves

as a cyst close to the tear; it has to be described as parameniscal cyst formation. In this case, treatment often involves partial meniscectomy.

Meniscal Tear, Indirect Signs

When a case is doubtful or has technical limitations, indirect signs may improve the reader's diagnostic accuracy. There are MR findings that may be associated with meniscal tears, and they have high specificity and high PPVs for an underlying tear. The most frequent signs include a parameniscal cyst, meniscal extrusion, and the shiny corner sign (see lemmas).

Meniscal Tear, Longitudinal

These tears occur in posterior horns in younger patients after significant trauma. At MR imaging, it appears as a vertically oriented line of high signal intensity perpendicular to the tibial surface and parallel to the long axis of the meniscus that divides the meniscus into central and peripheral halves (Fig. 3), without involvement of the free edge of the meniscus.

There is a close association between peripheral longitudinal tears of the LM and ACL tears. Because of the complex posterior attachments of the LM, it could be uneasy identifying its peripheral longitudinal tears of the posterior horn; anyway, it

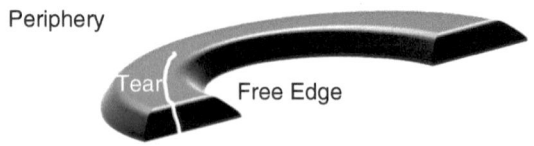

FIGURE 3 The scheme represents a longitudinal tear

may be useful to evaluate the integrity of the posterosuperior popliteomeniscal fascicle on T2-weighted MR images.

Meniscal Tear, Radial

Radial tears commonly involve the posterior horn of the MM or the junction of the anterior horn and body of the LM; tear is perpendicular to tibial surface and long axis of the meniscus, and its progression is from the free edge (avascular or "white zone" of the meniscus) to the periphery. Lesion is frequently not repaired (low healing). In contrast to horizontal and longitudinal tears, a radial tear has to be assessed first of all on axial MR images, which appear as "cleft" oriented perpendicular to the free edge. Various imaging signs can be seen with a radial tear, including the "truncated triangle," "cleft," "marching cleft," and "ghost meniscus" signs (see lemmas) (Figs. 4 and 5).

Meniscal Tear, Root

This is a radial tear of the meniscal root highly associated with meniscal instability and meniscal extrusion (more fre-

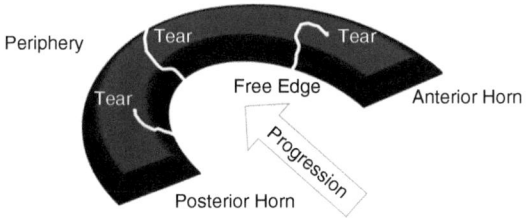

FIGURE 4 The scheme represents a radial tear. Take attention on the progression of the tear from the free edge (avascular or "white zone" of the meniscus) to the periphery

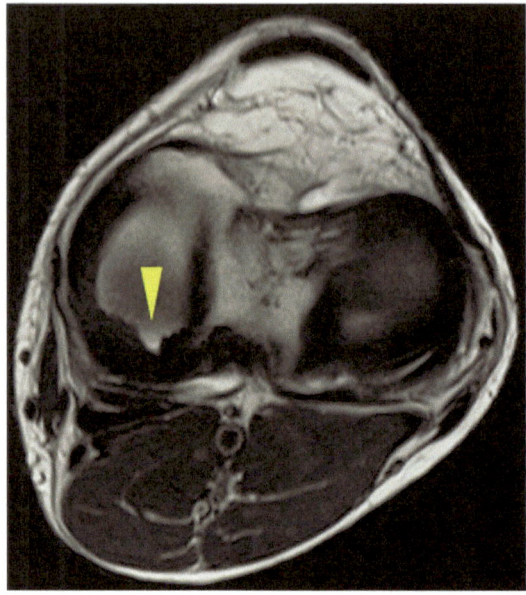

FIGURE 5 Radial tear opened: axial TSE T2-weighted image shows a radial tear progression perpendicularly to the C fibers of the meniscus (*arrowhead*)

quent on MM). This tear may be "underdiagnosed" if the meniscal root is not seen also in coronal planes (should course over its respective tibial plateau on at least one image) in fluid-sensitive MR images (magic-angle artifact). Lateral root tear is often associated with ACL tear and has to be suspected. Acute root tears without significant underlying degenerative changes are often promptly repaired because postoperative healing is facilitated by the adjoining rich synovial blood supply (Fig. 6).

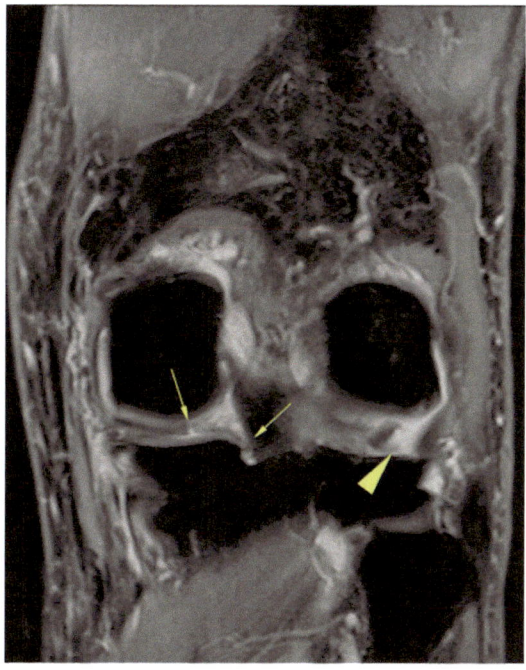

FIGURE 6 Meniscal root tear: coronal PD FS shows disruption of the posterior root of the medial meniscus with small radial lesion (*arrows*). Note the apparent absent lateral meniscus (*arrowhead*) that is a partial volume of fluid distension across the popliteus tendon

Meniscal Truncated Triangle

A truncated meniscus is defined as a truncation of the free edge, with preservation of its peripheral portion, often as a result of a partial-thickness radial tear.

Menisci, Variants

Meniscal tear may be mimicked by anatomic variants and pitfalls such as discoid meniscus, meniscal flounce, meniscal ossicle, and chondrocalcinosis. See lemmas in each sections.

Meniscocapsular Tear

This is a tear of the peripheral region of the meniscus at the menisco-synovial junction. It is more frequent for the posterior horn of the MM as its firmer contact with the joint capsule and the meniscotibial (coronary) ligament. MCS of the LM can arise at the superior or inferior popliteomeniscal fascicles near to the popliteus tendon and can result in meniscal instability with tear of the posterior horn. Healing is common because of the rich blood provision in the meniscal periphery and capsule.

- On MR, it is possible to appreciate an increase of distance between meniscus and capsule with interposition of articular fluid, best examined on fluid sensible images (sagittal and axial plane).

Meniscofemoral Ligaments

The meniscofemoral ligaments (MFLs) connect the posterior horn of the lateral meniscus with the lateral facet of the medial femoral condyle. The anatomy, the function, and the imaging of the MFLs are not well established among anatomists, orthopedics, and radiologists. The name of the third cruciate ligament and the name of ligament are not correctly used because MCF is not extended from a bone to another bone but from LM to a bone. It splits into two bands, anterior meniscofemoral ligament (ligament of Humphrey) and posterior meniscofemoral ligament (ligament of Wrisberg) in relation to PCL. The ligament is clear in MR coronal planes and in sagittal planes in which a tear of the posterior horn of LM has to be excluded (see Discoid Meniscus).

Meniscus, Postoperative

It can be difficult to interpret images of a meniscus after it was subjected to a surgical approach. When a partial meniscectomy is performed, some meniscal fragments are not evaluable in their anatomical location. In this case a careful patient history avoids errors and mistakes with a radial meniscal tear (see cleft sign of LM). In the case of meniscal suturing of a longitudinal lesion, a hyperintense tear is still visible in the sequences with short TR, and correct a diagnosis of re-rupture becomes tough. In this case it is appropriate to evaluate the tear on the sequences with long TR (fluid sensitive as DESS or TSE) in order to identify lesions of the surface of the meniscus in which the joint fluid enters. Finally we must not forget that the meniscal healing is often based on the arrangement of myxoid tissue that has high signal in both weighted images. Only in the latter case, in selected patients, it may be useful to administrate gadolinium, in which, on the contrary of a tear, the scar tissue presents significant enhancement.

MOAKS

MOAKS is based on a knee segmentation in 14 articular zones. Differently to BLOKS and WORMS, this score is more focused on articular BMLs also in subspinous regions. The patella is divided into medial and lateral, the femur into six medial and lateral anterior, central, and posterior zones and the tibia into six medial and lateral (anterior, central, and posterior) chondral zones plus the subspinous zone (tibial spines). It is should be better to use sequences as TSE T2-/intermediate-weighted or FS PD in the axial, coronal, and sagittal planes. When the patient is analyzed for the first time, immediately before chondral surgery, it is preferable to perform a 3D FSE as Cube (GE vendor) or SPACE (Siemens vendor), in order to obtain an accurate estimation of BMLs, best evaluable in the postsurgical follow-up. In the score, several articular features were evaluated:

- *BMLs*: these are ill-defined areas with low signal in sequences with low TR and hyperintense in sequences with high TR with surrounding well-defined areas of bone marrow cysts, with similar signal. This aspect is decisive in the OA evaluation because orthopedic surgeons need to know the size and depth of the chondral defect and in addition the "quality" of the subchondral bone and marrow that is essential for the correct integration of the chondral implants. BMLs must be graded as percentage of occupation in each knee zone (0 for none, 1 for <33%, 2 for 33–66%, and 3 for >66%). Osteophytes must be excluded in this phase.
- *Chondral layer*: cartilage defect must be scored both as percentage of occupation in each zone (size) and as percentage of full-thickness loss (depth).
- *Osteophytes*: these must be categorized on the basis of the size (extension from the joint rather than total volume) with 0 for none, 1 for small, 2 for medium, and 3for large.
- *Synovitis and joint effusion*: these are based on Hoffa's signal on sagittal images scored as 0 for normal, 1 for mild, 2 for moderate, and 3 for severe.
- *Menisci*: the score includes the typical features of a degenerated and damaged meniscus which are the anterior or medial/

lateral extrusion (on sagittal and coronal images 0 for <2 mm, 1 for 2–2.9 mm, 2 for 3–4.9 mm, and 3 for >5 mm) and the morphological changes as the presence of different type of lesions and tears (yes or no).

- *Ligaments and tendons*: ACL, PCL, and patellar tendon are graded on the basis of the presence of absence of lesions or partial lesion and a complete tear (0 or 1); the presence of associated bone remodeling and cysts are score as yes or no.
- *Periarticular features*: these are scored as the absence or presence of pes anserine, ITB, infrapatellar and prepatellar bursa inflammation, and popliteal and ganglion cysts.
- *Loose bodies*: these are scored as absent or present.

MOCART Score

The MOCART score is a system of evaluation for autologous chondrocyte implants. It may improve prospective multicenter studies with long-term follow-up of cartilage repair, also when different cartilage repair techniques are performed. The ideal superiority of the MR in the interpretation subchondral bone and bone marrow changes, on the contrary of arthroscopy, must be carefully considered above all when a three plane acquisition is performed, in order to avoid an underestimation of the chondral defect on images acquired. In the score, several articular features were evaluated:

- *Defect filling*: the margins of the defect must be the same of the native chondral layer (total or partial repair); the presence of the implant hypertrophy or exposure of the bone must be evaluated.
- *Border areas*: the integration with native chondral layer must be evaluated also on the border of the implant, and the

presence of fissures must be highlighted (particular attention to lateral fluid on the implant).

- *Quality of repair tissue layer*: implant's layer must be homogenous and fibrillation or irregularity must be excluded.
- *Structure of repair tissue layer*: clefts must be excluded.
- *Signal of repair tissue layer*: low intensity or iso-intensity in 2D or 3D FSE.
- *Status of subchondral lamina*: the signal of the interface between the implant and remodeled bone must be evaluated on the basis of signal on T1-weighted images as low signal intensity corresponds to low tropism of the bone lamina with poor prognosis for the implant integration and duration.
- *Subchondral bone features*: bone remodeling represents a poor prognostic aspect for implant integration as the presence of cysts, granulation tissue, and bone edema exposes the implant to the pressure on joint fluid which detaches the implant.
- *Joint effusion or inflammation*: abundant fluid in the joint beyond three months from the surgery must be carefully evaluated for the presence of implant hypertrophy or adhesions areas. This aspect correlates also with the persistence of pain symptom.

Suggested Reading

Bhatia S, LaPrade CM, Ellman MB et al (2014) Meniscal root tears: significance, diagnosis, and treatment. Am J Sports Med 42(12):3016–3030

Davis KW, Rosas HG, Graf BK (2013) Magnetic resonance imaging and arthroscopic appearance of the menisci of the knee. Clin Sports Med 32(3):449–475

Hunter DJ, Guermazi A, Lo GH et al (2011) Evolution of semi-quantitative whole joint assessment of knee OA: MOAKS (MRI Osteoarthritis Knee Score). Osteoarthritis Cartilage 19(8):990–1002

Nguyen JC, De Smet AA, Graf BK et al (2014) MR imaging-based diagnosis and classification of meniscal tears. Radiographics 34(4):981–999

Rosas HG (2014) Magnetic resonance imaging of the meniscus. Magn Reson Imaging Clin N Am 22(4):493–516

Runhaar J, Schiphof D, van Meer B et al (2014) How to define subregional osteoarthritis progression using semi-quantitative MRI osteoarthritis knee score (MOAKS). Osteoarthritis Cartilage 22(10):1533–1536

Wadhwa V, Omar H, Coyner K et al (2016) ISAKOS classification of meniscal tears-illustration on 2D and 3D isotropic spin echo MR imaging. Eur J Radiol 85(1):15–24

N

No lemma

M. Osimani, C. Chillemi, *Knee Imaging*, A-Z Notes in Radiological
Practice and Reporting, DOI 10.1007/978-88-470-3950-6_14,
© Springer-Verlag Italia 2017

O

Ogden Classification

This is the classification for tibial tubercle fractures, in six types. In type 1, there is a fracture of the distal portion of the tubercle without (1A) or with (1B) dislocation of the fragment; in type 2, there is fracture of the entire tubercle with separation from the tibia (2A) or with fragmentation (2B); in type 3, the fracture involves the tibial epiphysis without (3A) or with (3B) dislocation of the fragment. While in type 1, the treatment is conservative with immobilization; in types 2 and 3, screw fixation is required.

Osgood-Schlatter Syndrome

In this syndrome, a microtrauma intersecting the lower deep patellar tendon may lead to the avulsion of the cartilage or bone on tibial tuberosity. The disease is more frequent before 13–15 years in girls and 15–19 years in boys because the ossification

M. Osimani, C. Chillemi, *Knee Imaging*, A-Z Notes in Radiological
Practice and Reporting, DOI 10.1007/978-88-470-3950-6_15,
© Springer-Verlag Italia 2017

center of the tibial tubercle is already opened and the stresses placed on fibrocartilage by the quadriceps muscles via the patellar tendon lead to a "traction osteochondritis." One of the first clinical signs of OSs is a painful bump at the insertion of patellar tendon: this is due to chronic inflammatory stimuli inducing the formation of heterotopic bone. The assessment of the disease must be carried out with various imaging methods which allows the examination of different characteristics of the syndrome such as bone deformity through radiographs, disruption or follow-up of tendon through sonography, and a correct staging of the disease through MRI.

• *Radiographs*: These permit the evaluation of tibial tubercle entirety. For a proper diagnosis of OSs, it is necessary to assess in plain films the edema in the soft tissue, patellar tendon, and Hoffa's fat. As in children, the tibial tubercle composition has mostly fibrocartilage, at the beginning of the acute phase, it may be absent of any signs of disease. After 1–2 months of inflammation, thin bone nuclei of ossification may be evident at the tendon insertion. On adult patients (>16 years for female and >20 years for male), a nodular avulsed bony fragment may be seen (tibial ossicle). It is important to consider the presence of associated inflammation (also with MRI), in order to avoid damages on patellar tendon secondary to chronic impingement. If surrounding inflammation is absent, the appearance of irregular ossification tubercle may be valued as a normal variant.

• *Sonography*: It is useful in the evaluation of patellar tendon inflammation and the possible presence of heterotopic calcification. In OSs with avulsion fragment typically are found hypoechoic zone on soft-tissues with curvilinear and echogenic line.

• *MRI:* MR is important for the primary staging of the OSs, because changes in marrow edema may represent a key point for the prognosis of the condition in order to exclude a tibial tubercle avulsion. The inflammation must be always present for the correct diagnosis. Furthermore, relying on TSE T2-weighted sagittal, SE T1-weighted images (axial and sagittal) must be carefully reported: tendon fiber disruption, bone integrity, signal of tibial tubercle, and the presence of signal void areas.

Osteoarthritis Imaging

Imaging of OA is an emergent branch in the studies about the knee degenerative changes, because the orthopedic surgery has new approaches to the chondral defect with new strategies and new conservative therapies. In particular, it is very useful, also for the radiologist, to consider the OA not only as a chondral "wear and tear" pathology but as a "whole-organ" disarray regarding multiple joint structures. In this field the traditional approach to the OA using the radiographs seems to be unsatisfactory, and new advanced MRI technique must be familiarized by the modern radiologist in order to improve the standardization of the studies and the actual surgical approach to this multifactorial and multicompartment pathology. We explain the radiological approach by the Ahlbäck classification system and by the Kellgren and Lawrence system (see lemmas) and MRI approach by Outerbridge grading system; semiquantitative morphologic assessment, WORMS, BLOKS, and MOAKS; and compositional techniques (see lemmas).

Osteochondral Injury Staging System

This system of classification is based on arthroscopic surgery features for grading traumatic chondral or osteochondral lesions on MRI. It may be assessed on basic fat-saturated PD sequences in order to evaluate the stability and the size of the fragment to plan the surgery. In stage 1, the lesion is only cartilaginous and MRI shows the subchondral edema, while on radiographs, none cortical defect is manifested; in stage 2, there is a subchondral defect for a stabile fracture that is seen on MRI by a low-intensity rim in the inner edema with a osteopenia area in the radiographs; in stage 3, the fragment is disjointed but nondisplaced, and on MRI, a high intensity rim is evident around the fragment with radiolucency which may be evident under the fragment; in stage 4, the fragment is displaced and the joint effusion and the bone crater is well evident on MRI and radiographs. In the first phase, the fragment displaced is hyperintense because of its chondral and viable bone predominant component, but in the later phases, the fragment becomes hypointense for the predominant bone sclerosis and necrosis; in stage 5, the osteoarthritis changes become prevalent with extensive bone remodeling and possible meniscal damages.

Osteochondritis Dissecans, Imaging

OCD is a pathology that indicates the presence of an osteo-chondral fragment segmentation from the native subchondral bone. It may be divided on juvenile or adult type (growth plates opened or not), and the most frequent location is the lateral aspect of the medial femoral condyle. Because of this location, the most recognized etiology is the repetitive microtraumatism (above all in jumper sports); were recognized as others causes also ischemia, ossification anomalies and genetic aptitude. The juvenile type has a better prognosis because of better vascularization of epiphysis.

Imaging of the OCD must be performed in order to locate the osteochondral fragment, the healing or the dislocation potentiality.

- *Radiography*: On radiographs the fragment may be underdiagnosed as long as there is a complete separation of the osseous layer from the native bone. We suggest to "read" the trabecular architecture that have the tendency to be perpendicular in the epiphysis, so an osteochondral fragment may appear as a lucency in the epiphysis with a loss of the sharp cortical line of the surface. In this phase it is impossible to evaluate the stability of the fragment, so an MRI examination must be performed.
- *MRI*: MRI may highlight less evident or occult lesions on plain radiograms and CT. It is crucial to perform sequences focused on the cartilage morphology (see lemma) and subchondral signal (FS PD or DESS imaging) in order to assess lesion stability or instability. On MRI and OCD, focus appears as semilunar area of the bone with a different signal in comparison to the native bone. MRI complete assessment of OCD staging includes several features that must be described: (1) MRI characteristics of an unstable lesion include the presence of high signal-intensity line on the bottom of the fragment on T2-weighted sequences (Fig. 1). This is due to the entering of the joint fluid in the fracture from the native epiphyseal bone that increases the pressure and exposes to enlargement of the tear and detachment of the osteochondral lesion. One must distinguish from a line with similar signal on T2-weighted images that is granulation/scar tissue that represents a healing attempt of the bone. For these situations Gd injection may help for the correct diagnosis because the scar tissue shows positive enhancement on the contrary of the articular fluid. On doubtful cases, a repetition of the sequence after 15 min from the administration of the contrast and quite articular movement may be helpful as the articular fluid permits an indirect joint MR arthrography. We advise against joint direct Gd injection because any articular variation in pressure may be dangerous for lesion dislocation. Focal interruption of cartilage layer and the presence of cyst or edema beneath the lesion are also

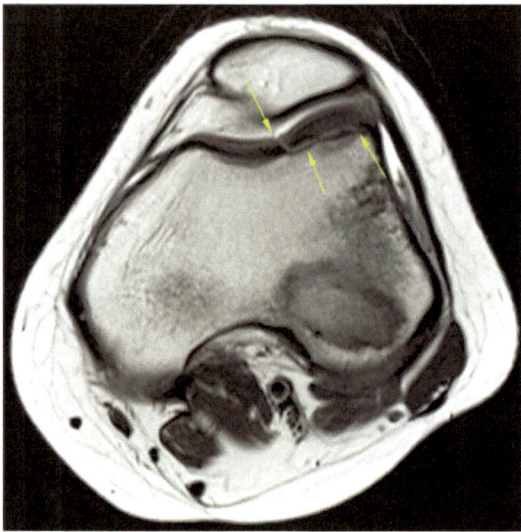

FIGURE 1 Chondral lesion not displaced: images show a chondral fragment not displaced on the external side of the femoral trochlea. The articular fluid demarcates the defect with an enlargement of the chondral layer
(*arrows*). This is a case of chondral defect with high risk of displacement.
Subchondral bone is quite intact (non-reabsorption areas)

indicating factors for potential detachment. (2) The signal of
the osteochondral fragment should be also carefully evaluated
on both T1-weighted and T2-weighted sequences in order to
assess the residual tropism of the fragment. A low signal on
both indicates poor vascular supplies with low healing and
high detachment potentiality. When a notch lesion is evident on
classical location of OCD, the detached fragment must be
excluded in the anterior synovial recess of the knee.
- *CT:* CT may be useful for the correct measurement of the
  osseous fragment and the bone notch, mostly when a surgery
  is required. The technique must be performed in conjunction
  with MRI examination.

Outerbridge Grading System

This is a classification based on arthroscopic surgery features for grading degenerative chondral defects on MRI. It may be valued on basic FS PD sequences and may be used both for patellar and femorotibial chondral defects. It is based on four grades: (1) the chondral layer shows hyperintensity with the absence of alterations; (2) chondral surface becomes quite irregular with fraying aspect; (3) focal ulceration becomes noticeable as partial lesions, without subchondral bone exposition; and (4) exposition and remodeling of the subchondral.

When OA is suspected, we suggest to use the MOAKS (see lemma) for grading other articular abnormalities.

Suggested Reading

Alizai H, Roemer FW, Hayashi D et al (2015) An update on risk factors for cartilage loss in knee osteoarthritis assessed using MRI-based semi-quantitative grading methods. Eur Radiol 25(3):883–893

Chen H, Xu W, Hu N et al (2015) antegrade drilling for unstable juvenile osteochondritis dissecans of the knee: mid-term results. Arch Orthop Trauma Surg 135(12):1727–1732

Chun KC, Kim KM, Jeong KJ et al (2016) Arthroscopic bioabsorbable screw fixation of unstable osteochondritis dissecans in adolescents: clinical results, magnetic resonance imaging, and second-look arthroscopic findings. Clin Orthop Surg 8(1):57–64

Ellermann JM, Donald B, Rohr S et al (2016) Magnetic resonance imaging of osteochondritis dissecans: validation study for the ICRS classification system. Acad Radiol 23(6):724–729

Giri S, Santosha, Singh CA, Datta S et al (2015) Role of arthroscopy in the treatment of osteoarthritis of knee. J Clin Diagn Res 9(8):RC08–RC11

Launay F (2015) Sports-related overuse injuries in children. Orthop Traumatol Surg Res 101(1 Suppl):S139–S147

Pascarella F, Ziranu A, Maccauro G (2015) Tibial tubercle fracture in a 14-year-old athlete with bilateral lower pole bipartite patella and osgood-schlatter disease. Case Rep Orthop 2015:815061

Penttilä P, Liukkonen J, Joukainen A et al (2015) Diagnosis of knee osteochondral lesions with ultrasound imaging. Arthrosc Tech 4(5):e429–e433

Rosa D, Balato G, Ciaramella G et al (2016) Long-term clinical results and
MRI changes after autologous chondrocyte implantation in the knee of
young and active middle aged patients. J Orthop Traumatol
17(1):55–62

Suzue N, Matsuura T, Iwame T et al (2014) Prevalence of childhood and adolescent soccer-related overuse injuries. J Med Invest 61(3–4):369–373

Tóth F, Nissi MJ, Ellermann JM et al (2015) Application of magnetic resonance imaging demonstrates characteristic differences in vasculature at
predilection sites of osteochondritis dissecans. Am J Sports Med
43(10):2522–2527

Yanagisawa S, Osawa T, Saito K et al (2014) Assessment of osgood-
schlatter disease and the skeletal maturation of the distal attachment of
the patellar tendon in preadolescent males. Orthop J Sports Med
2(7):2325967114542084

Yen YM (2014) Assessment and treatment of knee pain in the child and
adolescent athlete. Pediatr Clin North Am 61(6):1155–1173

P

Parameniscal Cyst

This is a pseudocyst rising from a meniscal tear wherein the
synovial fluid is entrapped. It is important to recognize a communication between the cyst and meniscal tear. This sign has a
PPV of more than 87 %, with the exception of the anterior horn
of the LM, where the PPV is near 65 %. Differential diagnosis
includes the articular ganglia, in which there isn't a communication with a meniscal tear (Fig. 1).

Parrot-Beak Tear

A parrot-beak tear is a progression of a radial and longitudinal
meniscal tear with displacement of the free edge. The tear is
correlated with knee mechanical locking or catching. In case of
a meniscal body abnormally small on sagittal images, it should

M. Osimani, C. Chillemi, *Knee Imaging*, A-Z Notes in Radiological
Practice and Reporting, DOI 10.1007/978-88-470-3950-6_16,
© Springer-Verlag Italia 2017

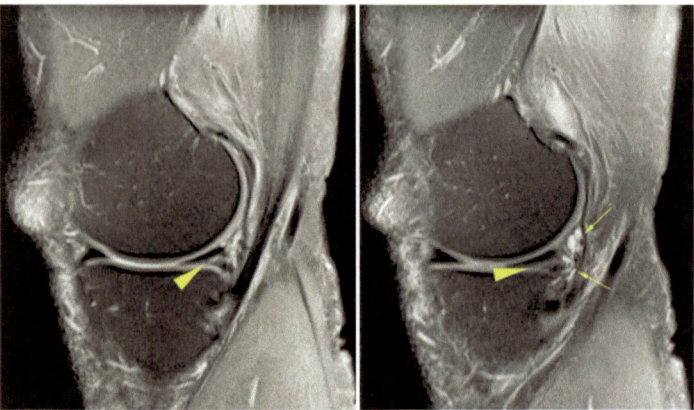

FIGURE 1 Parameniscal cysts: sagittal consecutive PD FS images (**a**, **b**) show medial meniscal oblique tear (*arrowhead*) with cystic fluid collection on the posterior margin of the meniscus (*arrows* on **b**); note that the posterior horn of the medial meniscus must be normally attached to the posterior capsule and a connection between tear a cyst may be seen on (**a**)

suspect a parrot-beak tear, and a careful search for a displaced fragment on axial planes must be performed (Fig. 2).

Patella Alta

In this condition, the patella is too high above the trochlear groove, due to long patellar tendon.

In patients with high-riding patella, the degree of flexion results too high for patellar engaging in the trochlea. When the knee presents a genu varum position, patella alta manifests itself because the extensor mechanism becomes the hypotenuse of a triangle, exposing the patella to subluxation. Patella alta may be measured on lateral radiographs or sagittal MR images with extended knee using the following:

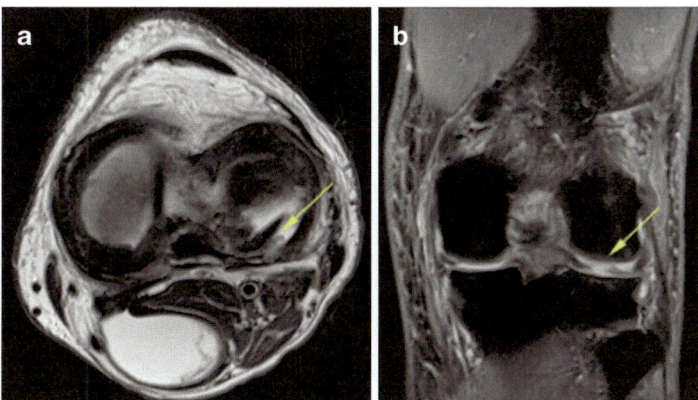

FIGURE 2 Displaced parrot-beak lesion: Axial TSE T2-weighted (**a**) and coronal PD FS (**b**) show a tear that combines features of a radial (perpendicular to C-shaped fibers) and longitudinal tear (parallel to C-shaped fibers). The result is the displacement of a meniscal portion similar to a parrot beak. Articular fluid into the lesion must be interpreted as instability feature of the tear (*arrows* in **a** and **b**). On coronal plane the meniscus seems absent. Abundant distension of the gastrocnemius-semimembranosus pseudo-bursa is also evident on axial plane

Patellar Tendon/Patella or Insall-Salvati Ratio

This is the ratio between the lateral height of the patella and the length of the patellar tendon (from the lower apex of the patella to the tibial tuberosity); a ratio >1.50 indicates a patella alta, while a ratio < 0.70 indicates a low patella (Fig. 3).

Patellar Delayed Ossification

This is a component of a syndrome known as nail-patella syndrome. This is an autosomal dominant ectodermal disorder affecting several organs with patellar hypoplasia, fingernail dysplasia, posterior iliac exostoses, and dysplasia of the radial

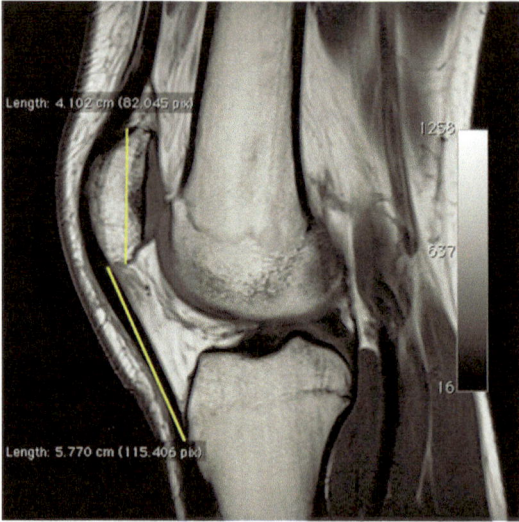

FIGURE 3 Insall-Salvati ratio: on the basis of measures on the image, the knee has an Insall-Salvati ratio of 4.1/5.7=0.71, compliant with "normal patella"

heads. The condition should be suspected when the patient does not extend the knee completely and radiographs show a small and luxated patella or even a patellar aplasia.

Patellar Fractures

Patellar fractures account for 1 % of total knee fractures and are classified according to bone exposure presence and fracture trace characteristic. Both aspects influence their treatment and management. The main types of patella fractures include vertical, marginal, transverse, and osteochondral fractures. The most common fracture is the transversal one. Separate diagnostic, imaging, and management processes and considerations are applicable to each type.

- *Radiography*: Radiograms are the most useful imaging modality in the majority of cases, with complications of a patellar fracture frequently identified radiographically. Anteroposterior (AP), lateral, and tangential or Merchant views should be featured in a radiographic examination for patellar fractures. In evaluating the trabecular pattern of the patella, comminution, and separation of fracture fragments, lateral views may be useful. In the assessment of vertical fractures and differentiating a fracture from a partitioned patella, tangential views are useful. Patella fractures may be obscured by AP radiographs. Radiology reports should note any distance over 3 mm between fragments of fractured patellar, as this may indicate increased incidence of posttraumatic degenerative arthritis and malunion. The identification of an osteochondral fracture is also crucial, as a loose body may occur if a fragment that contains cartilage, subchondral bone, and trabecular bone is displaced. In transverse fracture, it is important to evaluate the fragment displacement. Osteochondral fragments are best demonstrated on the lateral view; usually it is possible to identify the presence of an effusion and a high-riding patella. Radiographs are less useful than other modalities (e.g., MRI) in characterizing any cartilaginous injury associated with an osteochondral patellar fracture and can define fractures not otherwise detectable by radiographic examination. Sleeve fractures are located in the coronal plane of the patella, and are difficult to diagnose with radiographs. Differentiating between acute fractures from a partitioned patella may pose challenges on radiographs. The features of bipartite patella include even, corticated, opposing margins, best seen in the tangential projection. Comparison of two knees may be useful.
- *CT*: CT is useful particularly when a suspected fracture cannot be seen on radiographs and for osteochondral injuries. If the CT scan results are normal, then a fracture can be

excluded. The use of CT scanning can prevent delays in treatment and identify the location of fragments and the position of any intra-articular loose bodies. CT scanning has limited usefulness in evaluating soft tissue and bone marrow injury, and an MRI should be considered. CT scans may be better than MRIs in identifying loose bodies. CT scans are obtained with the patient in the supine position and with 15° of external rotation of feet pressed against a footrest at 90°. A complete exam comprises three scans with the knee resting, extended quadriceps contracted, and with a flexion of the knee of 15° with a relaxed leg. Multiplanar reconstruction should be done to better localize the displaced fragments. CT cannot determine the age of fractures because it may remain evident for up to 24 months.

- *MRI*: MRI may have to be used as a complementary exam. Actually it can identify abnormalities not evident on radiographs or where clinical diagnosis is difficult, as in patients with sleeve fractures as well as soft tissue and bone marrow injury. To assess all the anatomic structures, several planes are necessary, so the minimal protocol needed is three planes, FSE T1 weighted and FSE T2 weighted or DP weighted fat saturated or short-tau inversion recovery (STIR). With MRI, it is possible to demonstrate edema and hemorrhage as areas of increased signal intensity on T2-weighted fat-saturated, DP-weighted fat-saturated, and STIR images. In case of quadriceps injuries, coronal planes are useful to evaluate the extension of the trauma. Muscular atrophy is better demonstrated by the use of T1-weighted imaging. With MRI, it is possible to distinguish cartilage posterior-lateral surface defect of the patella from osteochondral pathology because of the absence of bone marrow alteration signal and the presence of a centimeter of well-defined area of intermediate/low signal on the T1 weighted.

Patellar Instability

Patellar instability is defined as the loss on physiological congruence between patellar and trochlear surfaces. This is a condition with an incidence of about 80/100000 subjects, more frequent in young women (second decade). It is meaningful to consider that patellar dislocation has a very high recurrence after the first episode of subluxation because of anatomical variants; activity and extensor mechanism damages develop a vicious circle and may lead to severe femoral-patellar OA, also in young patients.

The knowledge of normal anatomy and anatomic anomalies of the extensor mechanism is crucial because the suspicions of primary cause of chronic instability must be reported for correct surgical/conservative treatment.

Patellar Instability, MRI Checklist After Patellar Dislocation

Patellar displacement represents a very common trauma in young adult, above all during sport activities. In these patients, it is often difficult to perform a clinical test because of pain and their reduced motility. Therefore it is crucial, in imaging report, to evaluate and describe several typical signs referred to the mechanism of luxation and the stabilizers' damages, to support the surgeon in the best therapeutic choice (conservative or surgical). Below we suggest a list of features that should be evaluated on MRI:

- *MFPL damages*: this is the first check to evaluate on axial T2-weighted images; it is appropriate to describe the precise location of damaged fibers on the basis of the location near the patella (retinacula) or near the MCL. To avoid misdiagnosis, it is important to heed to the associated vastus medialis damages. Partial or complete disruption appears as soft tissue edema with or without low-signal fibers. On the basis of partial or complete disruption of MFPL, the patella typically may not return to its normal position, even after reduction, and patellar tilt may represent a helpful sign for MFPL disruption.

- *Patellar defects*: during the lateral dislocation, the patella leaves out the trochlea and the quadriceps tendon keeps the medial patellar surface on the lateral surface of the external condyle. The resultant bone to chondral bone impact causes a bone bruise area with focal edema of subchondral bone. In this case it is appropriate to examine carefully the chondral layer of the medial patella region to check if there is delamination of cartilage due to tangential forces, with more or less involvement of the subchondral bone (chondral or osseous-chondral fracture). The correct diagnosis of this condition is crucial because larger lesions (>1 cm^2) or displaced fragments should be surgically operated.

- *Lateral condyle defects*: on the other side of the impact, the lateral condyle may display edema, with more sporadic thin low-intensity rim representing an intracortical fracture (T1-weighted images).

- *Joint effusion*: it is not specific for the patellar dislocation, but a fluid depth >4 mm into the patellar recess and >8 mm in the lateral recess is suggestive for anterior compartment damage. When the fluid is very profuse, and the capsule is disrupted, it is important to evaluate fluid leakage zones on the extra-articular tissues, indicating a complete capsule lesion. When fluid-fluid levels are recognized, a concomitant lesion of the vastus medialis should be suspected.

Patellar Shape, Wiberg Classification

This is a classification based on the visual measure of asymmetry between lateral and medial patellar facets. It may be estimated on axial radiographs or MRI. The grading of the classification corresponds to grading of the asymmetry. In detail we may consider three grades: (1) the more "functional" patella in which the facets are symmetrical and equally sized with concave shape; (2) medial facet is quite smaller than the lateral that maintains a concave shape; (3) the medial facet is virtually absent with vertical orientation. The third shape is often presented together with flattened trochlea and patella hyperpressure on the lateral side; this aspect predisposes to patellar subluxation/instability.

Pes Anserine

This is a group of sartorius, gracilis, and semitendinosus conjoined tendons with insertion onto the proximal medial tibia superficially to the medial collateral ligament. It has a deep bursa that is distal and anterior to the medial collateral ligament bursa. The anatomical position of the bursa is useful to distinguish a pes anserine bursitis from other fluid collections of the posteromedial knee. A MCL bursitis is located in the medial side of the MCL, while a meniscal cyst generally is located inside the capsule or between the three layers of the capsule. When a meniscal tear is evident, the main diagnosis has to be a meniscal cyst also when a communication is less evident. A semimembranosus or tibial collateral ligament bursitis shows a "horseshoe" appearance of the fluid collection around the semimembranosus tendon.

PCL Avulsion Fracture

This injury involves PCL avulsion at insertion with the tibia and is difficult to diagnose only by clinical signs. The trauma mechanism is characterized by leg hyperextension or anterior direct force applied to the tibia.

- *Radiography*: This injury may present as discontinuity of the posterior tibial articular surface, usually seen best in the lateral view.
- *MRI*: Due to high detection accuracy, MR is the standard in assessing the fracture and the extent of damage, as well as chondral surfaces, meniscal tears, and other ligaments. The injury may be seen as a bone fragment attached to an otherwise intact PCL and separated from the remainder of the tibia. The edema and the surrounding soft tissues infarction may conceal the true dimension of the fragment. Particular attention must be also carried out on the T1-weighted signal of the fragment, above all in chronic lesions, as the fracture may lead to necrosis of the fractured bone.

Popliteomeniscal Ligaments

The popliteomeniscal fascicles arise from popliteus musculo-tendinous junction to the peripheral posterior horn of the LM and make a "tunnel" for the popliteus tendon to pass from an intra-articular to an extra-articular location. The resulting popliteal hiatus is shaped by two bands of popliteomeniscal fascicles: the anteroinferior and the posterosuperior fascicles. Rarely it is possible to recognize a third fascicle: the posteroinferior popliteomeniscal fascicle.

Posterior Cruciate Ligament, Anatomy

The PCL arises from the articular facet of the medial femoral condyle with a flat upper portion and a convex lower segment. The tibia attachment is on the posteroinferior recess of the tibial plateau. The ligament is 40 mm in length and 15 mm in width. Like the ACL, the PCL is intra-articular but extra synovial. Some authors considered the PCL as a ligament complex with the meniscofemoral ligaments (see lemma).

Posterior Cruciate Ligament, Imaging

- *Radiography*: The technique is used in order to exclude avulsion fractures or hemarthrosis and to evaluate the posterior tibial displacement, like in ACL tears.
- *Computed tomography*: Computed tomography (CT) may be useful to highlight an avulsion fracture of tibial attachment, mostly with three-dimensional reconstructions.
- *Magnetic resonance*: MRI is the gold standard imaging for PCL tears and very often associated capsular lesions. It is a specific protocol performed with a small FOV (10–16 cm) with a matrix of 256 or better and two excitations and 4 mm of slice thickness. Spin-echo techniques are preferred. On images, PCL appears as homogeneous low-signal bundles, except near the femoral insertion, where some hyperintensity may be seen on T2-weighted images. Magic-angle artifact is less present in comparison to ACL, because of more linear tendency of fibers, so the sagittal plane may be confidently used for diagnosis of a tear.

Posterior Cruciate Ligament, Tear

A striated appearance is the first feature indicating a ligament tear, above all, in the intraligamentous type. When a partial tear is present, it is possible to associate this feature with a ring of high signal in T2 (edema) or also on T1 images (hemorrhage).

Ligament disruption is often located in tibial insertion, with bone marrow edema and a bony fragment on a retracted ligament. Chronic tear of PCL appears as low signal of the ligament, and may be difficult to differentiate from a partial tear. Helpful signs of biomechanical incompetence of the ligament are an enlarged ligament, a serpiginous course, and insertion bone remodeling. It is relevant to remember that hardly ever a lesion of PCL is isolated, as relationship with capsular (MCL or LCL), ACL, or meniscal lesions is very often remarkable.

Posterior Oblique Ligament

This is the ligament forming the posteromedial aspect of the knee capsule from the second and the third layers according to Hughston. It has three distal insertions on posterior surface of the tibia, on posterior capsule and the oblique popliteal ligament, and on the semimembranosus tendon. Its biomechanical function is to support the dynamic role of the semimembranosus tendon.

Suggested Reading

Bistolfi A, Massazza G, Rosso F et al (2011) Non-reducible knee dislocation with interposition of the vastus medialis muscle. J Orthop Traumatol 12(2):115–118. doi:10.1007/s10195-011-0134-2

Chen HN, Yang K, Dong QR et al (2014) Assessment of tibial rotation and meniscal movement using kinematic magnetic resonance imaging. J Orthop Surg Res 9:65

Cowden CH 3rd, Barber FA (2014) Meniscal cysts: treatment options and algorithm. J Knee Surg 27(2):105–111

Gwinner C, Märdian S, Schwabe P et al (2016) Current concepts review: fractures of the patella. GMS Interdiscip Plast Reconstr Surg DGPW 5:Doc01

Park JH, Ro KH, Lee DH (2012) Snapping knee caused by a popliteomeniscal fascicle tear of the lateral meniscus in a professional Taekwondo athlete. Orthopedics 35(7):e1104–e1107

Pedersen RR (2016) The medial and posteromedial ligamentous and capsular structures of the knee: review of anatomy and relevant imaging findings. Semin Musculoskelet Radiol 20(1):12–25

Tigchelaar S, Rooy J, Hannink G et al (2016) Radiological characteristics of the knee joint in nail patella syndrome. Bone Joint J 98-B(4):483–489

Q

Quadriceps Myotendinous Strain

Through MR images, it is possible to assess tendon damages due to an overstretch of the myotendinous and distal insertion of the quadriceps muscle group. At first grade an interstitial edema is appreciated on T2-weighted FS sequences compatible with stretch injury and minimal fibers disruption; at second grade the edema is also hyperintense in T1-weighted images according to hematoma for partial fiber lesions and bleeding; on third grade there is a total fiber lesion with muscle retraction and abundant hematoma. Radiographs or sonography may be used for excluding the presence of calcification in the repair phase of partial rupture (myositis ossificans).

Quadriceps Tendon Avulsion Fracture

Avulsion fracture of the quadriceps tendon is uncommon and is related to strong deceleration caused by strong and abrupt contraction of quadriceps muscle with flexed knee. Quadriceps

M. Osimani, C. Chillemi, *Knee Imaging*, A-Z Notes in Radiological Practice and Reporting, DOI 10.1007/978-88-470-3950-6_17,
© Springer-Verlag Italia 2017

tendon avulsion is clinically evident but must be confirmed by imaging.

- *Radiography*: It is possible to detect this fracture by lateral view revealing comminuted bone fragments stemming from the superior aspect. Also an abnormal low patellar position can be detected. In chronic avulsion microcalcifications are noticed within the torn tendon.
- *MRI*: *MR* sagittal views may reveal that the distal quadriceps tendon has separated from the superior patella and marrow edema in the upper patellar pole; it is better seen in fat-suppressed long TR imaging like STIR or PD imaging.

Suggested Reading

Grando H, Chang EY, Chen KC et al (2014) MR imaging of extrasynovial inflammation and impingement about the knee. Magn Reson Imaging Clin N Am 22(4):725–741

Melville DM, Mohler J, Fain M et al (2016) Multi-parametric MR imaging of quadriceps musculature in the setting of clinical frailty syndrome. Skeletal Radiol 45(5):583–589

Yablon CM, Pai D, Dong Q et al (2014) Magnetic resonance imaging of the extensor mechanism. Magn Reson Imaging Clin N Am 22(4):601–620

R

Reverse Segond Fracture

A reverse Segond fracture is the opposite of the Segond one occurring as a result of external rotation and abnormal valgus stress, characterized by avulsion of distal tibial insertion of the MCL. Because of the trauma mechanism, these fractures are associated with disruption or avulsion of PCL as well as medial meniscal tears.

- *Radiography*: This fracture appears as an elliptic bone fragment on the medial articular surface of the proximal tibia.
- *MRI*: In cases of suspected reverse Segond fracture, an MRI should be undertaken to determine the extent of any associated injuries including tears to the medial meniscus and PCL injuries.

M. Osimani, C. Chillemi, *Knee Imaging*, A-Z Notes in Radiological Practice and Reporting, DOI 10.1007/978-88-470-3950-6_18, © Springer-Verlag Italia 2017

Suggested Reading

Engelsohn E, Umans H, Difelice GS (2007) Marginal fractures of the medial tibial plateau: possible association with medial meniscal root tear. Skeletal Radiol 36(1):73–76, Epub 2006 Mar 29

Escobedo EM, Mills WJ, Hunter JC (2002) The "reverse Segond" fracture: association with a tear of the posterior cruciate ligament and medial meniscus. AJR Am J Roentgenol 178(4):979–983

Peltola EK, Lindahl J, Koskinen SK (2014) The reverse Segond fracture: not associated with knee dislocation and rarely with posterior cruciate ligament tear. Emerg Radiol 21(3):245–249

S

Salter-Harris Fractures

Salter-Harris fractures involve the growth plate of long bone in pediatric patients (children between 10 and 15 years old). These fractures are classified regarding what structures are involved, the physis or metaphysis or epiphysis. Accurate classification of the injury is crucial; indeed the fracture can compromise the normal mechanism of endochondral ossification with formation of the bone bridging through the growth plate or damage the proliferation zone in the epiphysis, causing premature closure of the physis with limb shortening or abnormal growth. Classification of SH fractures is based on nine types of fractures. Types I–V are the most common. To remember the most frequent types, use the mnemonic SALTR (slipped, above, lower, through/transverse/together, ruined/rammed).

- *Imaging*: In cases where fracture is suspected, radiography in AP and lateral view is the preferred preliminary modality, and findings will vary depending on the type of injury. However, radiographic examination may be difficult if the injury is serious and the patient is in acute pain and unable to

M. Osimani, C. Chillemi, *Knee Imaging*, A-Z Notes in Radiological Practice and Reporting, DOI 10.1007/978-88-470-3950-6_19, © Springer-Verlag Italia 2017

be positioned correctly. In such circumstances, it may be beneficial to further evaluate the injury with CT scanning after the plain radiographs have been evaluated if radiographic findings are inadequate. CT shows tomographic multiplanar information and bone detail, and MRI shows marrow edema and abnormal bone bridging of the physis and may assess areas of abnormal bone trophism due to the fracture. MRI must be performed in patients with doubtful radiograms.

Segond Fracture

Segond fracture is due to avulsion fracture of the iliotibial band, fibular collateral ligament, and biceps femoris tendon and can be seen on MRI examination or anteroposterior radiographs.

Semimembranosus Tendon Avulsion Fracture

This specific type of avulsion injury to the semimembranosus tendon involves external rotation and abduction of flexed knee or abnormal varus stress, mechanisms that happen usually in athletes.

- *Radiography*: This fracture is difficult to detect radiographically and may be seen only in lateral view as a displaced bone fragment posterosuperior from its insertion on the tibia.
- *MRI*: In cases where this fracture is suspected, further investigation with MR imaging is warranted to investigate possible associated injuries including posterior meniscocapsular separation, medial posterior horn meniscal tear, and anterior cruciate ligament disruption.

Shiny Corner Sign

The term has the same meaning of ankylosing spondylitis seen
on MR and represents the appearance of peripheral bone marrow lesions. This may be considered as an indirect sign of
meniscal instability after a root tear.

Sinding-Larsen-Johansson Syndrome

Differently from OSs, this syndrome affects the proximal insertion of the patellar tendon on the patella.

These two syndromes share a similar etiology in fact repetitive
microtraumatisms, especially during jumping sports, lead to the
definition of the same condition in adults as "the jumper's knee."

- *Radiographs*: On plain films the edema in the prepatellar soft
  tissue and patellar tendon effusion may be observed.
  Ossification into the proximal tendon may also represent a
  diagnostic feature, with a blurred appearance of the cortical
  surface of the inferior pole on the patella.
- *MRI*: MR is important for the differential diagnosis of tendon
  rupture, in which the abnormal signal is seen only into the
  proximal tendon, while the edema in true Sinding-Larsen-
  Johansson syndrome is seen also in the inferior pole of the
  patella. MR images are also useful for the follow-up and staging of related inflammation of surrounding soft tissue and
  prepatellar bursa (Fig. 1).

Speckled Lateral Meniscus

This is a possible pitfall and it cannot be mistaken with a tear of
anterior horn of LM. The speckled appearance can be seen as a

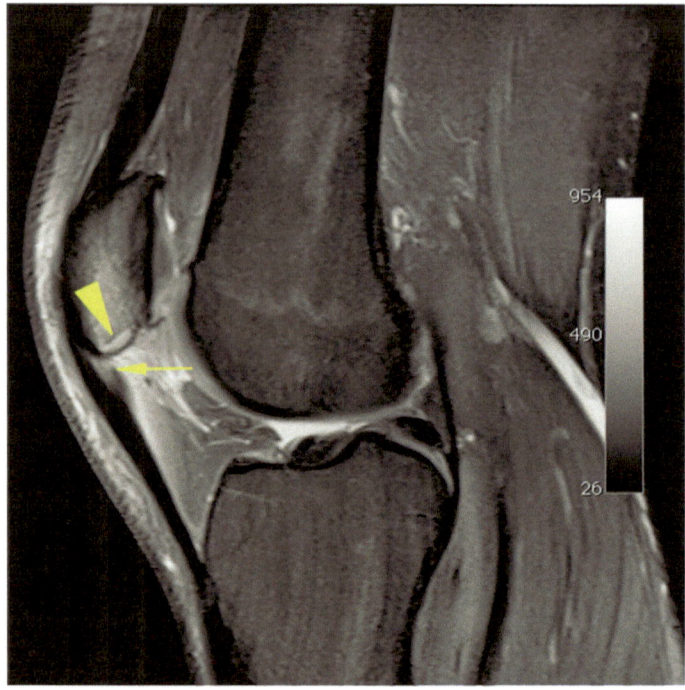

FIGURE 1 *Sinding-Larsen-Johansson*: PD FS sagittal image shows abnormal signal on the proximal patellar tendon (*arrow*) with quite edema on the inferior pole of the patella (*arrowhead*). Inflammation of surrounding soft tissue and prepatellar bursa are also evident

normal variant of anterior horn of LM, and it is due by fibers of the ACL inserting into the meniscus.

- MRI: The anterior horn of LM shows a speckled-like appearance.

Suggested Reading

Chauvin N, Jaramillo D (2012) Occult distal femoral physeal injury with disruption of the perichondrium. J Comput Assist Tomogr 36(3):310–312

Draghi F, Danesino GM, Coscia D et al (2008) Overload syndromes of the knee in adolescents: sonographic findings. J Ultrasound 11(4):151–157

Gottsegen CJ, Eyer BA, White EA et al (2008) Avulsion fractures of the knee: imaging findings and clinical significance. Radiographics 28(6):1755–1770

Hill BW, Rizkala AR, Li M (2014) Clinical and functional outcomes after operative management of Salter-Harris III and IV fractures of the proximal tibial epiphysis. J Pediatr Orthop B 23(5):411–418

Iwamoto J, Takeda T, Sato Y et al (2009) Radiographic abnormalities of the inferior pole of the patella in juvenile athletes. Keio J Med 58(1):50–53

McKenna SM, Hamilton SW, Barker SL (2013) Salter Harris fractures of the distal femur: learning points from two cases compared. J Investig Med High Impact Case Rep 1(3):2324709613500238

Suzue N, Matsuura T, Iwame T et al (2015) State-of-the-art ultrasonographic findings in lower extremity sports injuries. J Med Invest 62(3–4):109–113

Valentino M, Quiligotti C, Ruggirello M (2012) Sinding-Larsen-Johansson syndrome: a case report. J Ultrasound 15(2):127–129

Van Dyck P, Vanhoenacker FM, Gielen JL et al (2010) Three-Tesla magnetic resonance imaging of the meniscus of the knee: what about equivocal errors? Acta Radiol 51(3):296–301

T

Tibial Tubercle Avulsions

In teenager, especially during jumping sports, it is frequent to see tibial tubercle fractures.

The OSs is one of the predisposing conditions, but with the absence of previous symptoms, it is not indicative for diagnosis. *Radiographs* are helpful for the diagnosis and correct staging according to the Ogden classification of tibial tubercle fractures.

Tibial Plateau Fractures

Tibial plateau fractures, also known as bumper fractures, are caused by axial loading, lateral, or twisting injuries. These fractures are associated with soft tissue involvement such as ACL on collateral ligament injuries that can compromise the articular stability resulting in posttraumatic osteoarthritis degeneration. The fractures are classified on the basis of condyles involvement and by the presence of articular surface

M. Osimani, C. Chillemi, *Knee Imaging*, A-Z Notes in Radiological
Practice and Reporting, DOI 10.1007/978-88-470-3950-6_20,
© Springer-Verlag Italia 2017

depression. Three classification methods are identified: Schatzker, OTA/AO, and Hold. Schatzker and OTA/AO are the most used. Depression fractures are most common in older patients and split fractures in younger.

- *Radiography*: Radiography exam is sufficiently accurate in the detection of tibial plateau fractures; however, nondepressed fractures can be overlooked. AP projection, cross table lateral, sunrise view, and oblique views are recommended if this fracture is suspected. In case of severe fractures, cross table lateral and AP may be the only choice. In such cases, the presence of lipohemarthrosis can suggest articular surface impairment.
- *CT*: CT scans have a key role in confirming and assessing complex fractures, in particular the relationship between bone fragments and anatomic structures, or assessing the involvement of articular surface with precision. For a clear image, the thickness of the scan needs to be 1 mm or less, allowing MPR reconstruction. It is possible that some fractures will be undetected with the use of only axial reconstruction images; however coronal and sagittal reconstructions may avoid this problem.
- *MRI*: The level of usefulness of MRIs in tibial plateau fracture management is still being studied. MRI is better in visualizing fracture patterns as well as full tissue injuries like meniscal injuries and certain ligament injuries than CT scans except in cases where the fracture was comminuted.

Trochlear Dysplasia

Trochlear dysplasia is defined as the anomalous morphology of the trochlea which is straight proximally with decreased concavity distally. The variant is considered as a developmental anomaly even because it often affects both knees. In some, severe, cases the trochlear surface develops into a convex shape because of prevalent hypoplasia of the medial condyle. This condition leads to loss of patellar tracking on the trochlea during the knee flexion and must be assessed on images.

Radiographs and CT

On lateral films, a normal trochlea presents sulcus crossing the anterior surfaces of the condyles also known as "the crossing sign"; instead if there is medial hypoplasia, it is possible to appreciate the "double contour sign" that is an abnormal double line of the anterior surfaces of the condyles. According to Dejour classification, we may consider four morphologic types of trochlear dysplasia: (1)"V" shape of the trochlea but less deep (sulcus angle of more than 150°), (2) flattened trochlea, (3) asymmetric oblique trochlea for medial condyle hypoplasia (Fig. 1), and (4) asymmetric oblique trochlea with vertical link between medial and lateral condyles (cliff pattern).

- *MRI*: Axial and sagittal planes may be used for trochlear morphology evaluation suitably when an axial radiogram is not available. In particular, some trochlear measures may be performed on MRI, and its variation may be assessed also during quadriceps contraction, with GRE images at suitable signal to time ratio, and the knee is 20° flexed.

    - *Lateral trochlear inclination*: For this measure the axial image with most salient trochlea is selected, and two lines are drawn on the subchondral bone of the trochlea lateral facet and behind the femoral condyles; the angle formed must be an inclination of more than 11°.
    - *Trochlear facet asymmetry*: This is the ratio between lateral and medial facet length; a trochlear ratio <0.4 is according to trochlear dysplasia.

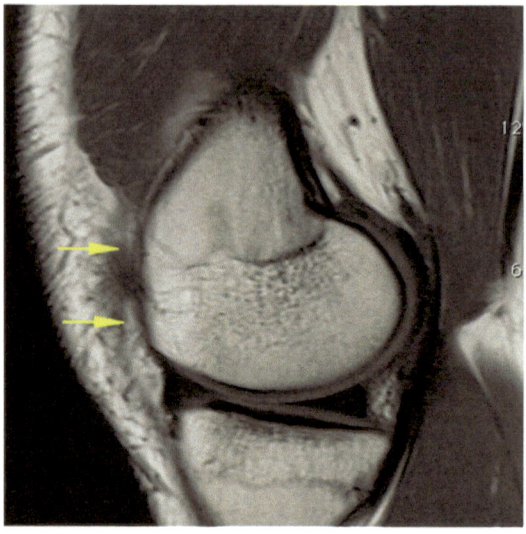

FIGURE 1 Trochlear dysplasia: Sagittal T1-weighted image shows medial condyle hypoplasia (*arrows*) as trochlear type 3 according to Dejour classification

- *Trochlear depth*: In this measure a reference line behind subchondral bone of condyles is plotted; three perpendicular lines are drawn, respectively, on the most salient point of lateral and medial facet and the deepest point of the femoral sulcus. A normal sulcus must have a greater depth of > 3 mm.
- *Trochlear groove angle*: This measure is obtained by the intersection of two lines drawn on the subchondral bone of highest point of the lateral and medial trochlear facet; the resultant angle must be included from 125° to 145°. Further, in the measures of trochlear dysplasia, it is important to report also the relationship of the trochlea with the inclination of the patella, so it is convenient to report other measures as (Fig. 2):

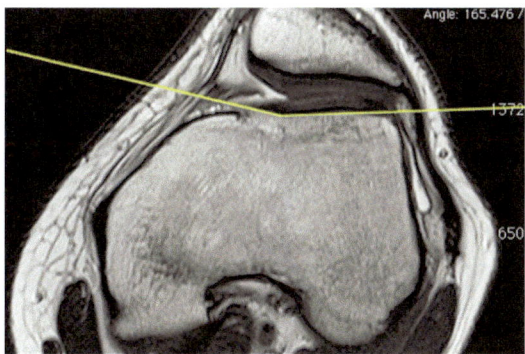

FIGURE 2 Trochlear groove angle: This is an example of flat trochlea with groove angle >145° (165°). Note that the lines must be drawn on the subchondral bone of the lateral and medial trochlear facet

- *Femoral-patellar congruence angle*: This represents the quantification of lateral subluxation of the patella; it is calculated from the angle formed by the line bisecting the trochlear groove angle and a line drawn from the apex of the patella to the apex of trochlear sulcus; the angle must be included in −8°±6°.
- *Patellar tilt angle*: This is the resultant angle between a line drawn behind the subchondral bone of the condyles and the lateral patellar facet. The normal angle is >8°. It is newsworthy to assess this angle before and after quadriceps contraction, in order to prove a lateral patellar hyper-pressure, due to extensor tendon asymmetry (see TT-TG Measure) (Fig. 3).
  - *Laurin angle*: This measure is obtained by drawing a line on the lateral patellar facet and the other on the anterior aspect of the trochlea; the resultant angle must be laterally opened with values from 8° to 15°. In lateral patella subluxation is expected. An angle is opened medially (Fig. 4).

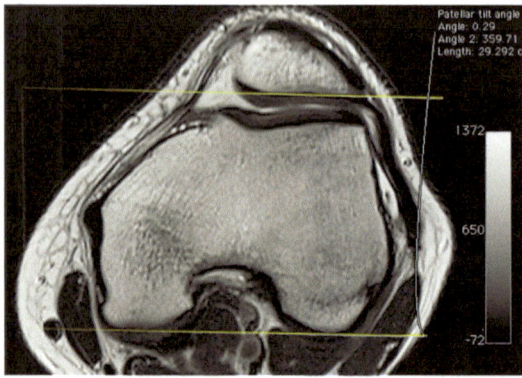

FIGURE 3 Patellar tilt angle: The normal angle is >8°. In this patient the resultant angle is 0.89 compliant with lateral patellar hyper-pressure

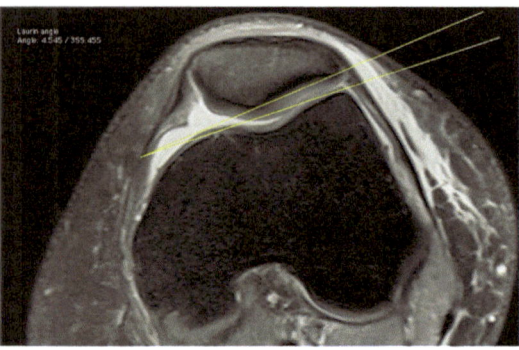

FIGURE 4 Abnormal Laurin angle: The PD FS image shows a laterally opened Laurin angle of 4.5°. This is compliant with later patellar hyperpression

TT-TG Distance

The tibial tubercle represents the fulcrum in which the patellar tendon, the lateral and medial patellar stabilizers, and the quadriceps tendon unload the forces during knee flexion. Therefore, so that the patella maintains a vertical alignment during flexion, the knee should ideally have the tibial tubercle aligned vertically to the femoral trochlea. A lateral tibial tuberosity exposes the patella to lateral displacement during the flexion, especially when the patella or the femoral trochlea has some morphological features that increase the risk of lateral displacement (see Trochlea and Patella Dysplasia). This is more glaring in young sportive in which the quadriceps contraction and the sport gesture can expose to traumatic patellar displacement. All the aspects described above may be summarized conceptually by the term of patellar maltracking and must be assessed in the radiographs or MR report, to avoid chondral resultant damages. The TT-TG is the measure of the lateralization of the tibial tubercle with respect to the trochlear groove; it is obtained overlaying two axial slices (CT or MRI), passing through the apex of the femoral sulcus and the tibial tubercle. On femoral slice a reference line is drawn behind the condyles, and two perpendicular lines must be drawn passing the apex of the trochlea and the tibial tubercle. The resultant distance between these lines must be <20 mm.

Suggested Reading

Frosch KH, Schmeling A (2016) A new classification system of patellar instability and patellar maltracking. Arch Orthop Trauma Surg 136(4):485–497

Hinckel BB, Gobbi RG, Kihara Filho EN et al (2016) Why are bone and soft tissue measurements of the TT-TG distance on MRI different in patients with patellar instability? Knee Surg Sports Traumatol Arthrosc

Kim HS, Yoo JH, Park NH et al (2016) Magnetic resonance imaging findings in small patella syndrome. Knee Surg Relat Res 28(1):75–78

Saffarini M, Demey G, Nover L et al (2016) Evolution of trochlear compartment geometry in total knee arthroplasty. Ann Transl Med 4(1):7

Song EK, Seon JK, Kim MC et al (2016) Radiologic measurement of Tibial Tuberosity-Trochlear Groove (TT-TG) distance by lower extremity rotational profile computed tomography in Koreans. Clin Orthop Surg 8(1):45–48

Weber AE, Nathani A, Dines JS et al (2016) An algorithmic approach to the management of recurrent lateral patellar dislocation. J Bone Joint Surg Am 98(5):417–427

Yi M, Hong SH, Choi JY et al (2015) Femoral trochlear groove morphometry assessed on oblique coronal MR images. AJR Am J Roentgenol 205(6):1260–1268

U

No lemma

M. Osimani, C. Chillemi, *Knee Imaging*, A-Z Notes in Radiological
Practice and Reporting, DOI 10.1007/978-88-470-3950-6_21,
© Springer-Verlag Italia 2017

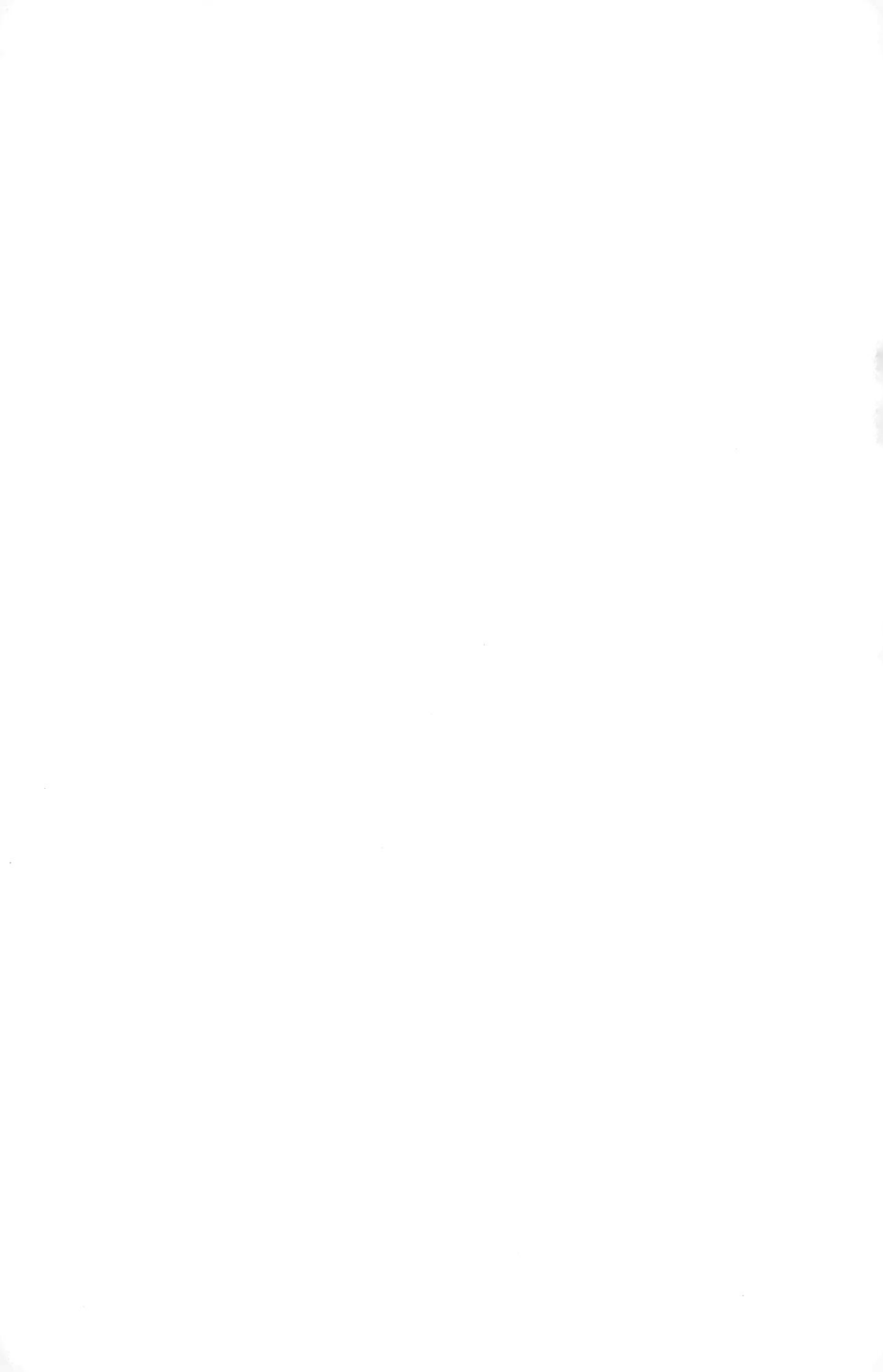

V

No lemma

M. Osimani, C. Chillemi, *Knee Imaging*, A-Z Notes in Radiological   119
Practice and Reporting, DOI 10.1007/978-88-470-3950-6_22,
© Springer-Verlag Italia 2017

W

WORMS

This is a semiquantitative score calculated on a cartilage segmentation on 15 or 6 areas. Images are scored on the basis of 14 articular structures and features: cartilage, bone marrow, subchondral cysts, bone remodeling and marginal osteophytes, menisci, cruciate ligaments, collateral ligaments, synovitis, loose bodies, and periarticular cysts/bursae. We report cartilage section of the score that is calculated on the basis of signal and morphology changes: 0 point assigned for the absence of signal or morphological changes on cartilage areas; (1) increased signal with fluid-sensitive intermediate-weighted sequences (see lemma Cartilage, Semiquantitative Morphologic Assessment); (2) partial-thickness chondral defect width < 1 cm, 2.5, full-thickness chondral defect width < 1 cm; (3) several areas of partial-normal thickness defects intermixed with areas of normal thickness or a partial-thickness defect more extensive than 1 cm but less than 75 % of the region; (4) diffuse loss of chondral layer ($\geq$75 % of the region); (5) multiple areas with full-

M. Osimani, C. Chillemi, *Knee Imaging*, A-Z Notes in Radiological
Practice and Reporting, DOI 10.1007/978-88-470-3950-6_23,
© Springer-Verlag Italia 2017

thickness defects (grade 2.5) or a full-thickness defect wider than 1 cm but less than 75 % of the region; and (6) diffuse (≥75 % of the region) full-thickness defects.

Wrisberg Variant, Discoid Meniscus

It represents the least common subtype of discoid meniscus (see lemma). In the Wrisberg variant, there is the absence or the thinning of posterior coronary ligament (see lemma) and capsular attachments resulting in more mobility of the LM, occasionally subluxing into the joint. Patients describe a snapping sensation during flexion or extension. Despite the typical clinical history, arthroscopy is nevertheless required for a definitive diagnosis of the Wrisberg variant. A Wrisberg variant should be wanted whenever a discoid meniscus is identified on MRI as the surgical approach, above all partial meniscectomy vs. repair it by providing a posterior attachment.

- *MRI*: Wrisberg LM should be difficult to find on MR images. The unique specific sign is the absence of normal fascicles and coronary ligaments that would normally attach the posterior horn of the lateral meniscus to the joint capsule and tibia. This aspect may be found with high T2 signal between the LM and the capsule and simulating a peripheral tear of posterior horn (LM may also sublux anteriorly).

Suggested Reading

Felson DT, Lynch J, Guermazi A et al (2010) Comparison of BLOKS and WORMS scoring systems part II. Longitudinal assessment of knee MRIs for osteoarthritis and suggested approach based on their performance: data from the osteoarthritis initiative. Osteoarthritis Cartilage 18(11):1402–1407

Jose J, Buller LT, Rivera S et al (2015) Wrisberg-variant discoid lateral meniscus: current concepts, treatment options, and imaging features with emphasis on dynamic ultrasonography. Am J Orthop (Belle Mead NJ) 44(3):135–139

Singh K, Helms CA, Jacobs MT, Higgins LD (2006) MRI appearance of Wrisberg variant of discoid lateral meniscus. AJR Am J Roentgenol 187(2):384–387

X

No lemma

M. Osimani, C. Chillemi, *Knee Imaging*, A-Z Notes in Radiological   125
Practice and Reporting, DOI 10.1007/978-88-470-3950-6_24,
© Springer-Verlag Italia 2017

Y

No lemma

M. Osimani, C. Chillemi, *Knee Imaging*, A-Z Notes in Radiological   127
Practice and Reporting, DOI 10.1007/978-88-470-3950-6_25,
© Springer-Verlag Italia 2017

Z

No lemma

M. Osimani, C. Chillemi, *Knee Imaging*, A-Z Notes in Radiological   129
Practice and Reporting, DOI 10.1007/978-88-470-3950-6_26,
© Springer-Verlag Italia 2017